Knowledge, Attitudes, and Perceptions of Preeclampsia among First-Generation Nigerian Women in the United States

Dr. Christine Okpomeshine

Order this book online at www.trafford.com
or email orders@trafford.com

Most Trafford titles are also available at major online book retailers.

Printed in the United States of America.

ISBN: 978-1-4907-2302-0 (sc)
ISBN: 978-1-4907-2304-4 (hc)
ISBN: 978-1-4907-2303-7 (e)

Library of Congress Control Number: 2013923805

Trafford rev.   01/06/2014

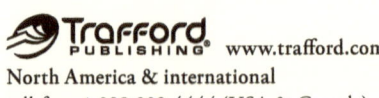

www.trafford.com
North America & international
toll-free: 1 888 232 4444 (USA & Canada)
fax: 812 355 4082

Table of Contents

List of Tables

List of Figures

Abstract

Although numerous studies have documented the need for early recognition and treatment of preeclampsia to attain a good prognosis, first-generation Nigerian women living in the United States tend to seek obstetrical care after the first trimester (12 weeks), by which time prompt recognition may be missed. The purpose of this study was to measure the knowledge, attitudes, and perceptions about preeclampsia and limitations that determine the delay in seeking obstetrical treatment in early pregnancy among first-generation Nigerian women living in the United States. This cross-sectional quantitative study consisted of 180 first-generation Nigerian women in the United States recalling their experiences of being diagnosed with preeclampsia and experiencing preeclampsia. The health-belief model served as the conceptual framework to predict the health behaviors of first-generation Nigerian women regarding their experiences in early recognition of signs and symptoms of preeclampsia. Data were collected through an online survey and analyzed using binary and ordinal logistic regression. The results indicated no statistical significance relation between knowledge, attitudes and perceptions of preeclampsia and demographic characteristics, socioeconomic status, acculturation, and access to healthcare. Despite the nonsignificance, these findings will help women better understand how to make positive health decisions and support the efforts of public health departments to produce and distribute a booklet on preeclampsia to all healthcare providers regarding the importance of early detection. This study contributes to positive social change by bringing awareness of preeclampsia, risk factors, and the need for early recognition and prompt treatment to first-generation Nigerian women living in the United States.

Dedication

This dissertation is dedicated to my family, religious sisters (Handmaids of the Holy Child Jesus), and friends. I would like to thank them for their patience, assistance, and support during the past few years. In addition, I dedicate this dissertation to my sister, Rosaria Downes, SC, and father, Lawrence Frizzell, who motivated me to continue my education. Finally, I dedicate this dissertation to my head nurse, Kathleen Giretti, RN, and friends. I hope that they will be mindful of the need to work hard to accomplish their goals and will be inspired to lead healthy and productive lives. I thank everyone for the overwhelming support that has been extended, and I am proud to share this momentous achievement with every person who has been a part of my journey.

Acknowledgments

Many individuals provided support during the course of preparing this doctoral dissertation and I would like to thank each of them. First, I must acknowledge Dr. Amany Refaat, my committee chairperson, for her inspiration and insight. She offered guidance and suggestions to keep the process on track. I also appreciate the insight of my committee member, Dr. Patrick Tschida, who provided suggestions to help improve my work and contribute to the success of my investigation. I would also like to thank Dr. Vincent Abgboto and Dr. Sherer for their assistance in reviewing my work and providing various forms of resources. Finally, I would like to thank all of the first-generation Nigerian women who participated in the study for their time and openness in sharing their preeclampsia experiences. To God is the glory.

CHAPTER 1

Introduction to the Study

Preeclampsia is the leading cause of perinatal morbidity and mortality (LaMarca, Gilbert, & Granger, 2008). Preeclampsia affects between 5 and 7% of pregnancies in the United States and 10% in Nigeria (American College of Obstetrics and Gynecology [ACOG], 2010). There have been numerous research efforts on the etiology of preeclampsia, risk factors, and treatment, but few studies on preventive strategies. Preeclampsia is one of the more common complications seen in obstetrics and has led to many maternal and perinatal deaths (Fisk & Atun, 2009). Preeclampsia occurs after the first trimester of pregnancy, with symptomology that includes elevated blood pressure, proteinuria, and edema of the face, hands, and feet (Levine & Lindheimer, 2009 Mothers' symptoms usually start at 20 weeks and disappear within 6 weeks of delivery, leaving mothers with major long-term complications such as cardiovascular disease and premenopausal period (Lain & Roberts, 2002). When preeclampsia is not treated promptly, it can lead to severe complications for the fetus and the mother (Centers for Disease Control and Prevention [CDC], 2007).

However, with proper treatment, the prognosis is encouraging and fetal complications can be largely avoided if the condition is controlled. Women who have risk factors for preeclampsia have increased chances of experiencing the condition but not necessarily having preeclampsia (CDC, 2007). Additionally, having no risk factors is not a sign that one will not have preeclampsia.

According to Lim and Steinberg (2010), the incidence of preeclampsia in healthy, nulliparous (first time) women ranges from 2 to 6% in the United States, whereas worldwide incidence accounts for 5 to 14% of all pregnancies, although in developing countries it ranges from 4 to 18% and is the second highest obstetric cause of preterm labor, preterm birth, and neonatal death (Backes et al., 2011). The most common complications of preeclampsia include premature placental separation in about 3 in 100 incidents of preeclampsia; blood clotting in about 3 in 100; and eclampsia (seizures) in about 2 per 100 (ACOG, 2010; Bhattacharya & Campbell, 2005; Osungbade & Ige, 2011).

In northern Nigeria, preeclampsia accounts for 40% of maternal deaths due to poor access to prenatal care, history of hypertension in pregnancy, multiple pregnancies, molar pregnancy, diabetes mellitus, and renal diseases (Abubakar, Abdullahi, Jibril, Dauda, & Poopol, 2009). Other causes of preeclampsia in northern Nigeria are socioeconomic factors such as poverty, poor obstetric healthcare-seeking behavior, lack of knowledge, cultural perceptions of preeclampsia and eclampsia, and lack of access to high technology during pregnancy, labor, the postpartum period, and newborn care (Abubakar et al. 2009). Preeclampsia and eclampsia are public health issues in the United States and worldwide. Even though efforts to minimize and cure the complications of preeclampsia have been recorded, additional steps need to be taken to achieve the preventive goal.

Problem Statement

Preeclampsia is a life-threatening complication of pregnancy and a debilitating disease for women. Preeclampsia impacts the social and economic life of pregnant women. In developing countries, in particular, many women lose their lives during pregnancy, childbirth, and the postpartum period because of preeclampsia. Early recognition and prompt treatment of preeclampsia are essential components of prenatal care. Pregnant women with preeclampsia should be educated about the complications and the importance of follow-up care. Not all healthcare facilities are equipped with skilled professionals and technology with the ability to assess and address preeclampsia.

Among the many studies on preeclampsia, very few have been conducted in Nigeria, and none were found among first-generation Nigerian women living in the United States. Although research has provided evidence of the extent of the disease, a gap exists among first-generation Nigerian women diagnosed with preeclampsia living in the United States.

Purpose of the Study

In this quantitative study, I assessed knowledge, attitudes, and perceptions of preeclampsia among first-generation Nigerian women living in the United States from their perspective and reviewed their understanding of early recognition of preeclampsia. The study was designed to address the gap in the literature and advance the body of knowledge regarding preeclampsia in first-generation Nigerian women living in the United States who were diagnosed with preeclampsia. The results of this study may remedy the misinformation acquired from mothers, grandmothers, aunts, and mothers-in-law, thus improving the educational standard of preeclampsia among this group of women. Finally, this study allowed first-generation Nigerian women living in the United States to share their experiences of preeclampsia and clarify their doubts regarding the disease process, offering a chance to document their ancestral beliefs on paper. These women related their understanding and gained additional knowledge of the preeclampsia they experienced, which may influence their decisions to seek early prenatal care in their next pregnancy. This learning took place while assessing the present and potential risks of women with a history of the disease.

Nature of the Study

In this quantitative study with a cross-sectional survey design, I assessed the relationship among knowledge, attitudes, perceptions, cultural beliefs, education, socioeconomic status, acculturation, and technology among first-generation Nigerian women living in the United States and preeclampsia. The sample was 180 first-generation Nigerian women selected from a purposeful sampling. These women completed an online SurveyMonkey survey. In an effort to explain the problem statement, the study was integrated with the health-belief model (HBM; Glanz, Rimer, & Lewis, 2002).

Research Questions and Hypotheses

Research Question 1: Is there a relationship between demographic characteristics, cultural beliefs, socioeconomic status, acculturation, and access to health care and knowledge of preeclampsia among first-generation Nigerian women with a history of preeclampsia living in the United States?

*H*a: Demographic characteristics, cultural beliefs, socioeconomic status, acculturation, and access to health care will be significantly related to knowledge of preeclampsia among first-generation Nigerian women with a history of preeclampsia living in the United States, as measured by attitudes questionnaire.

*H*0: There is no relationship between demographic characteristics, cultural beliefs, socioeconomic status, acculturation, and access to health care and knowledge of preeclampsia among first-generation Nigerian women with a history of preeclampsia living in the United States.

Research Question 2: Is there a relationship between demographic characteristics, cultural beliefs, socioeconomic status, acculturation, and access to health care and attitudes of preeclampsia among first-generation Nigerian women with a history of preeclampsia living in the United States?

*H*a: Demographic characteristics, cultural beliefs, socioeconomic status, acculturation, and access to health care will be significantly related to attitudes of preeclampsia among first-generation Nigerian women with a history of preeclampsia living in the United States.

*H*0: There is no relationship between demographic characteristics, cultural beliefs, socioeconomic status, acculturation, and access to health care and attitudes of preeclampsia among first-generation Nigerian women with a history of preeclampsia living in the United States.

Research Question 3: Is there a relationship between demographic characteristics, cultural beliefs, socioeconomic status, acculturation, and access to health care and perceptions of preeclampsia among first-generation Nigerian women with a history of preeclampsia living in the United States?

*H*a: Demographic characteristics, cultural beliefs, socioeconomic status, acculturation, and access to health care will be significantly related to perceptions of preeclampsia among first-generation Nigerian women with a history of preeclampsia living in the United States.

*H*0: There is no relationship between demographic characteristics, cultural beliefs, socioeconomic status, acculturation, and access to health care and perceptions of preeclampsia among first-generation Nigerian women with a history of preeclampsia living in the United States.

Conceptual Framework

The conceptual framework demonstrates how theories inform the research (Leshem & Trafford, 2007). There were many variables in this study (parity, gravidity, weight, diet, education, cultural beliefs, technology, acculturation, socioeconomic status, access to health care, and problems of the trophoblast) (Kanayama, 2003). Conceptually, a framework describes the reason for the study design and method used to collect data (Leshem & Trafford, 2007). Many key factors relate to preeclampsia among first-generation Nigerian women, according to the reviewed literature. The goal of this study was to measure the experiences of preeclampsia among this target population. One conceptual model was used to create a framework and evaluate data.

According to Denison (1996) and Lennon (2005), the HBM describes important guidelines for actions that might positively impact adherence to health-prevention programs geared to prevent, control, treat, or alleviate health problems. Focusing on the experiences of these pregnant women may enhance preeclampsia detection. This model consists of perceived susceptibility of contracting a disease such as preeclampsia, whereas perceived severity refers to the belief that the disease will be fatal. Perceived benefits are individual adherence to health promotion and prevention to prevent the disease; self-efficacy refers to the confidence acquired to perform health-related activities. Finally, cues to action refer to any strategy that brings awareness in controlling the progression of a disease. HBM explains the readiness of women to change health-related beliefs, participate more in health screenings and prevention programs, and educate others about preeclampsia.

For this critical public health challenge, multifaceted interventions have been found to be effective (Grol, 2001). These interventions require a combination of several ways to promote patient teaching and guidance: increase awareness of primary, secondary, and tertiary preventions; provide direct and indirect care of patients; develop strategies to help patients remember appointments; and create incentives for adequate follow up. According to Johnson et al. (2006), the focus of HBM is to overcome limitations through the delivery of categorized interventions for many people, those willing and those unwilling to change.

HBM provides a concept that triggers individuals to decide to remain healthy and avoid unpleasant results (Rosenstock, Strecher, & Becker, 1988). Because preeclampsia poses danger in pregnancy, pregnant women ideally may want to prevent preeclampsia by using elements of healthcare guidance that will trigger healthy decision making and result in desirable outcomes. According to Becker (1974), individuals have changed their health beliefs because of HBM (see Figure 1).

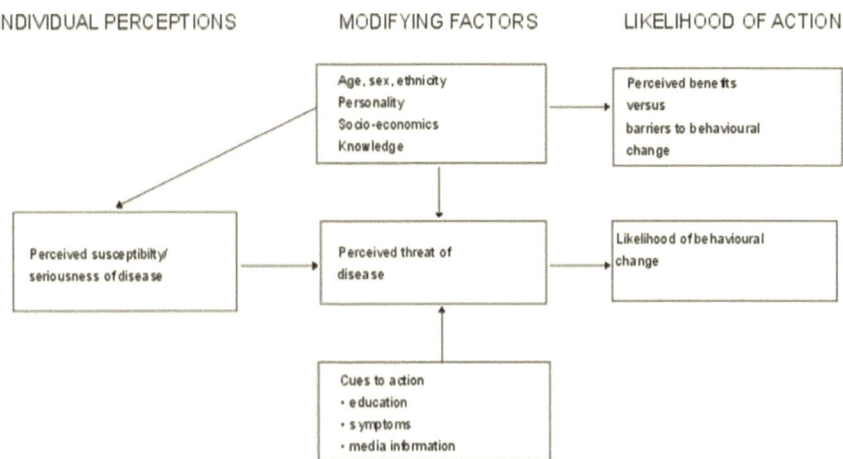

Figure 1. Health belief model. From *Health Behavior and Health Education: Theory Research and Practice,* by K. Glanz, B. K. Rimer, & F. M. Lewis, 2002, San Francisco, CA: Wiley & Sons, p. 52. Used with permission (see Appendix A).

According to Li et al. (2009), barriers to healthcare use in the United States are divided into three categories, ranging from accessibility to care, to knowledge, to attitudes and beliefs about the healthcare system. According to Li et al., the use of the HBM creates an avenue to health promotion and education while bringing awareness to prompt health-seeking behavior. Because first-generation Nigerian women's beliefs about early prenatal care do not address the issue of preeclampsia well, the HBM is a good model for this study.

Implications for Positive Social Change

As a result of this study, an increasingly broad body of knowledge regarding preeclampsia in first-generation Nigerian women living in the United States may be achieved. There may be an increased understanding of the disease process, bringing awareness of early recognition and treatment to decrease disability. According to the Institute of Medicine (1988), the mission of public health is to fulfill the "community's interest in assuring conditions in which people can be healthy" (p. 3). This study ensured that women could be healthy giving birth, free from the complications of preeclampsia. The findings from this study may help move the public health field closer to minimizing complications of preeclampsia among women, thus preventing deaths in pregnancy, labor, and the postpartum period.

Definition of Terms

Abruptio placentae: Also known as placental abruption; refers to the separation of a placenta after the 20th week of gestation and prior to birth (Gaufberg, 2011).

Gravidity: Number of times a woman has been pregnant (Creinin & Simhan, 2009).

Hypoxemia: Low oxygen in the blood and decreased maternal tissue blood flow preceding preeclampsia. Hypoxemia may cause one to experience shortness of breath (Karanam, Page, & Anim-Nyame, 2010).

Molar pregnancy: An abnormal form of growth (hydatidiform mole) in the uterus that mimics pregnancy but does not have a fetal heartbeat (National Center for Biotechnology Information, 2010).

Oliguria: A decreased urine output of less than 30ml in an hour and 400ml in a day (Devarajan, 2008).

Proteinuria: A condition of an abnormal amount of protein in the urine. One of the most frequent causes of nephritic syndrome in pregnancy is the presence of proteinuria. Hence, it differentiates between preeclampsia and gestational hypertension. The excretion of large amounts of protein in the urine of two random samples 4 hours apart with a greater than normal amount of protein is significant (Hladunewich, Karumanchi, & Lafayette, 2007).

Thrombocytopenia: A disorder of an abnormally small number of platelets. Platelets help blood to clot; this disorder is associated with excessive bleeding (Nabili, 2009).

Assumptions

In this study, it was assumed the participants were honest in their answers and responded to the needs of this study. The study accommodated experiences shared and operated from the standpoint that the inquiry conforms to the health belief model conceptual framework used.

Limitations

There were potential limitations to this study.

1. Because the target population was in a specific location in New York City, the findings could not be generalized to other localities.
2. Purposive and convenient sampling could not be used to generalize to a large population of first-generation Nigerian women.

The dependent variable has more than two categories: ordinal logistic regression (proportional odds models) was used to investigate the relationship between the dependent variable and independent variables. When binary logistic regression was used, a problem arose of complete separation or quasicomplete separation; thus, not all the independent variables were included in all models.

Although quantitative research has been used for years, there is controversy regarding whether structural bias and generalization continue to manifest (Creswell, 2003; Ulin, Robinson, & Tolley, 2005). The data collection methods used in a particular quantitative study determine its structural bias and generalizability. In this study there were many possible variables, but only a subset of them was used to answer the research question. However, these were self-reported cases of preeclampsia with no clinical documentation sought to confirm diagnosis of this illness. Most cases of pregnancy-induced hypertension can be reported as preeclampsia because healthcare personnel generally associate any incidence of high blood pressure in pregnancy with preeclampsia.

The researcher anticipated a response rate of 130 (from the $N = 180$ participants) because the assumption was that participants from this population had Internet access and were willing to participate to the end of the study. Participants who did not have Internet access, had never been pregnant, and were not first-generation Nigerian women were disqualified from the study. The survey questions and methodology might have been biased.

Scope and Delimitations

The scope of this quantitative study was the experiences of first-generation Nigerian women, used to identify behaviors that support or hinder women's health during pregnancy. The delimitation was that participants in this study were limited to first-generation Nigerian women who were or were not pregnant; also, all participants were women. Therefore, Nigerian men and other African women were excluded from the population.

Summary

This chapter presented the mortality and morbidity of preeclampsia in the United States and among first-generation Nigerian women in the United States. In this chapter, I discussed the obstetrical benefits of recognition and prompt treatment of preeclampsia. The conceptual framework used in this study was the HBM. The research questions and hypotheses were applicable to assessing the knowledge, attitudes, and perceptions of preeclampsia among first-generation Nigerian women living in the United States.

Chapter 2 is a review of the literature offering a broad dissection of the instrument that was used in the study. Various theories that may predispose women to preeclampsia are discussed. The literature review compares and evaluates methodological approaches and results to bring awareness of risk factors of preeclampsia and the complications caused by delay in seeking early treatment.

Chapter 3 presents a review of the study's design and methods. This study used a quantitative approach to answer the research questions. The method of data collection was an Internet survey questionnaire of first-generation Nigerian women in the United States who had experienced preeclampsia. The choice of the research design and methods is justified.

Chapter 4 provides the results of the analysis, divided into (a) demographic description and findings, (b) information of variables used for proportional odds ratios, and (c) summary of the results. Data were collected through SurveyMonkey and analyzed with SPSS 17.0 for descriptive and inferential analysis. In Chapter 5, I interpret the findings and conclude with a summary, limitations, implications of positive social change, and a recommendation.

Cooper and Lawler (2001) described obstetrical accessibility in the United States as unequally distributed by number of healthcare providers, geography, and health insurance. This study adds to the continuing training for healthcare providers to upgrade skills in different disease specialties to improve quality of care; promote the rights and dignity of patients as well as healthcare providers; and develop leadership, accountability, and teamwork skills (Manongi, Marchant, & Bygbjerg, 2006).

CHAPTER 2

Literature Review

This chapter examines risk factors associated with preeclampsia in the United States. Many first-generation Nigerian women experience preeclampsia during the second trimester, which leads to a long-term hospital stay (Redman & Sargent, 2005). Despite this known danger in pregnancy, physicians have not been able to prevent preeclampsia. Although worldwide studies have been conducted on preeclampsia, no study has been conducted on first-generation Nigerian women in the United States.

This chapter includes an overview of preeclampsia, including related medical complications, statistics of impact, symptoms and diagnosis, and risks and guidelines for this medical condition. This section of the paper will describe the detection, theory of the processes, and education in counseling prevention, biomarkers, and studies on other population groups in Nigeria. It will include clinical presentations of other diseases associated with preeclampsia, various theories of the disease, increased pressor responses, prostaglandins, vascular endothelial growth factors (VEGFs), genetic and immunological factors, and inflammatory factors. The role of homocysteine and the placenta will also be included in this chapter.

The literature review will evaluate the body of research that investigated attitude and perceptions of preeclampsia among Nigerian women. This review will include many qualitative and quantitative studies that investigated knowledge-acquisition perceptions of preeclampsia among Nigerian women because there is no literature on first-generation Nigerian women living in the United States. The literature review will use numerous research studies and methods to ascertain the knowledge and healthcare accessibility of Nigerian pregnant women diagnosed before and after preeclampsia.

The methodology of the research design and decision of the instrumentation followed the guidance of the reviewed literature. The review of literature was conducted digitally through electronic searches in psychology, obstetrics, and medical databases. These included PsycINFO, PsycARTICLES, MEDLINE, CINAHL, Medscape, Cochrane Database of Systematic Reviews, Cochrane Pregnancy and Childbirth Group's Trials Register, EMBASE, and ProQuest, as well as the Walden University Library Database. The search terms were *preeclampsia, hypertension in pregnancy, blood pressure increase in pregnancy involving Nigerian women with preeclampsia and proteinuria,* and *eclampsia.* Preeclampsia was found in literature on African American, Caucasian, Latino, and Asian women and those in several African nations. Numerous books were used to gain an overview of preeclampsia.

Overview of Preeclampsia and Related Complications

Preeclampsia is a hypertensive disorder that presents with many complications distinctive to pregnancy. According to the CDC (2007), preeclampsia is a medical condition with a triad of increased blood pressure, protein in the urine, and edema, and happens in about 12 to 22% of pregnancies and 17.6% of maternal deaths in the United States. However, the terms and categories of this disorder are often misunderstood. A risk factor for growth retardation, hypoxemia, premature birth, and neonatal death is preeclampsia. The ACOG (2010) reported that preeclampsia is a serious danger to the lives of a mother and child and is the leading cause of maternal death. Generally, there are several adverse problems such as convulsions, *abruptio placentae,* disseminated intravascular coagulation, and cerebral hemorrhage related to women with preeclampsia. ACOG stated that it was important to develop effective treatment and prevention strategies with the goal of early recognition during pregnancy and also to identify individuals at risk. In most cases, the major cause of maternal mortality in the developed and the developing world are hypertensive disorders of pregnancies. Preeclampsia and hypertension in pregnancy are major public health concerns. However, treatments of pregnancy-induced hypertension and preeclampsia have not changed from their standards of care and medical care depends on an accurate diagnosis. The CDC documented that many researchers and public health leaders studied risk factors for ways to decrease resultant disabilities.

Statistics of Impact

According to ACOG (2010), rates of preeclampsia in the United States rose from 2 to 6% in healthy nulliparous women, whereas the rates rose 4 to 18% in developing countries. Preeclampsia is a major contributor to a poor pregnancy (ACOG, 2010). Tucker, Berg, Callaghan, and Hsia (2007) described preeclampsia as accounting for 2% of their study population. In that study, 33% were Hispanic, 29% were White, 26% were Black and foreign born, and 12% were Asian. Among the Black women, the rate for those with preeclampsia was 2.9%, Hispanic women were 2.6%, 1.3% were White, and Asian women 1.2%. Tucker et al. concluded the risk for preeclampsia was greater than that for obesity and excessive weight gain in pregnancy.

Symptoms and Diagnosis

Preeclampsia develops after 20 weeks of gestation (Lain & Roberts, 2002). Preeclampsia starts with defective development of the placenta and can endanger the lives of mother and child (Sebire et al., 2002). A hemolytic disorder—hemolysis, elevated liver enzymes, and low-platelet syndrome—is common in preeclampsia and also can be seen in other medical, surgical, and obstetrical conditions (Sibai & Stella, 2010). However, these conditions are associated with increased mortality during and after pregnancy. Most preeclamptic women who survive this debilitating condition may develop long-term complications. Sibai (2004) pointed out that differential diagnoses can be confusing because many diseases mimic preeclampsia laboratory and clinical findings. The clinical criteria used to diagnose preeclampsia are elevated blood pressure of 140 mmHg systolic or more, or 90 mmHg diastolic or more, or raised blood pressure after 20 weeks of gestation with previously normal blood pressure (Wagner, 2004). A 24-hour urine specimen with protein excretion of 0.3 g protein or higher, edema, visual disturbances, headache, and epigastric pain are all indicative of preeclampsia (Gangaram, Ojwang, Moodley, & Maharaj, 2005). Hemolysis, elevated liver enzymes, and low platelet counts are abnormalities seen in laboratory values (K. Khan, Wojdyla, Say, Gülmezoglu, & Van Look 2006; Rawashdeh, 2010). Two urine samples collected randomly at least 4 hours apart or diminished urine less than 500 ml in 24 hours may lead to adverse complications (Gangaram et al., 2005).

Preeclampsia complication with a new onset of *grand mal* seizures is recognized as eclampsia (Zeeman, Fleckenstein, Twickler, & Cunningham, 2004). There are other medical conditions that can cause seizures that are unrelated to pregnancy such as a bleeding malformation of artery and vein, bleeding in a large vessel, or idiopathic seizure disorder (Prahlow & Barnard, 2004). A superimposed preeclampsia criterion includes a sudden proteinuria elevation prior to 20 weeks of gestation; a sudden elevation in blood pressure; or having a hemolysis, elevated liver enzymes, and low-platelet syndrome counts (Wagner, 2004). Indications superimposed on preeclampsia of a patient with chronic hypertension are headaches or epigastric pain (Vigil-De Gracia, Montufar-Rueda, & Ruiz, 2003). The manifestations of severe preeclampsia were documented by Brichant, Dewandre, Foidart, and Brichant (2010) as proteinuria, hypertension, malfunction of the nervous system, liver trauma, decreased platelet and urine output, edema of the pulmonary vessels, cerebrovascular accident, and severe intrauterine growth restriction. Severe preeclampsia in pregnancy must be closely monitored in the hospital to make an accurate diagnosis and to control and stabilize progression of the disease.

Various Theories on Preeclampsia

According to Karanam et al. (2010), preeclampsia poses severe universal morbidity and mortality warnings for mother and fetus. Preeclampsia is known to affect about 2 to 3% of pregnancies with an unknown cause, but many theories relate to the origin of this pathology (ACOG, 2010). Pathologic findings indicate blood-pressure elevation was not a factor (Hirschi, 2000). Poor tissue perfusion leads to vasospasm and peripheral resistance (Karanam, 2003). According to Xiong, Demianczuk, Saunders, Wang, and Fraser (2002), women with preeclampsia and hypertension have larger babies than is normal at gestational age, contradicting the previous belief of uteroplacental insufficiency that causes small babies for their gestational age. There is a decreased perfusion effect in the mother and the fetus. Nevertheless, the authors concluded preeclampsia is hereditary and not easy to determine. However, there were pathological and hemodynamic changes in preeclampsia and pregnancy that induced hypertension. Powers et al. (2008) reported elevated maternal plasma in cellular fibronectin in preeclamptic women that led to intrauterine growth restriction. Preeclampsia also suggested the difference in races between angiotensinogen polymorphisms of the M235T gene seen in hypertension and preeclampsia and the AGT 217 gene in the angiotensinogen basal-promoter region. Shenoy, Kanasaki, and Kalluri (2010) revealed numerous associations between angiogenesis and metabolism with preeclampsia. They encouraged research in preeclampsia pathogenesis.

According to Munger, Van Tassell, and LaFleur (2007), the main reason for uncontrolled hypertension was noncompliance in about 50-75% of patients in antihypertensive treatment. Failure to adhere to this treatment was the most significant clinical problems in the care of hypertension. Thus, public health interest is to improve the treatment of hypertension. There are various theories leading to an understanding of preeclampsia. A metabolite known as homocysteine has been documented as causing endothelial cell dysfunction (Kulkarni et al, 2010). Many studies have examined the association between serum homocysteine concentrations and preeclampsia.

Koopmans et al. (2009) encouraged and recommended the induction of labor for all hypertensive pregnant women after 37 weeks of gestation. This action would reduce severe maternal morbidity and improve the maternal outcome. Similarly, Srinivas et al. (2009) suggested an association between chronic hypertension and babies who are small for gestational age and concluded that intrauterine growth restriction could be more prevalent in women with chronic hypertension who develop preeclampsia than those with original preeclampsia. Dorland (2010) revealed a complication of preeclampsia relating to the development of auditory processing in the fetus. Upon examination of the comparisons between spontaneous and auditorily elicited fetal behaviors from 33 to 39 weeks gestational period, there were no significant differences in behavioral auditory processing. Therefore, most documentation reflected complications seen in the fetus of mothers with mild to moderate preeclampsia, compared to mothers with normal pregnancies.

Studies on Preeclampsia

A study by Uboh, Ebong, Oton, Itam, and Barnaby (2008) indicated an increase in free radicals and decrease in the antioxidant vitamins found in 100 Nigerian women at 24 weeks gestation with preeclampsia. Also, a study by Shaarawy, Zaki, Ramzi, Salem, and El-Minawi (2005) showed that an increase in bone resorption and decreased bone formation were noted in preeclamptic mothers and their fetuses. Accurate diagnosis of pregnancy-induced hypertension and preeclampsia are achieved through effective strategies of care. In the same way, Jim, Sharma, Kebede, and Acharya (2010) described maternal and perinatal death worldwide as a result of severe preeclampsia and eclampsia.

A study presented by Swende and Abwa in 2009 also showed fundoscopic problems in severe preeclamptic women, revealing bilateral papilla edema and macular edema that responded to antihypertensive treatment, preventing seizure and a caesarean section after stabilization. The researchers found a relationship between endothelial cells and preeclampsia in pregnancy complicated with Lupus. Soluble fat-mobilizing substances, like tyrosine kinase, are also associated with preeclampsia and systemic Lupus (Levine et al., 2009). Eclampsia is an important contributor to mortality in low-income countries (Zeeman et al., 2004).

Biomarkers

Biomarkers such as calcium supplementation and a set of proteins have been identified as instrumental in potential screening tests for preeclampsia. In research carried out by Hofmeyr, Lawrie, Atallah, and Duley (2010) and a similar study by Vigeh et al. (2006), exposure to environmental metals such as lead, antimony, and manganese increased the risk of preeclampsia in women without occupational exposure. Vigeh et al. found that the placenta of patients with preeclampsia had calcification of the wall of the umbilical cord vessel and a high concentration of lipoproteins similar to atherosclerotic lesions in preeclampsia. Research initiated by Blumenstein et al. (2009) identified proteins in the blood of pregnant women that may predict the development of preeclampsia. Prior to developing this medical condition, these blood proteins were seen more often in those women who later became preeclamptic than in those women with normal pregnancy. Therefore, identifying these biomarkers will introduce the development of a potential screening test for preeclampsia (Maynard et al., 2010)

Increased Pressor Responses

A normal pregnancy develops refractoriness to infused vasopressors. In women with preeclampsia, there was an increased vascular reactivity to pressors (AbdAlla, Lother, EI Massiery, & Quitterer, 2001).

Woisetschläger et al. (2000) used either norepinephrine or angiotensin II. Kaaja et al. (2004); Spaanderman, Ekhart, de Leeuw, and Peeters (2004); and Vallotton (2008) used vasopressin. Kanagasabai (2010) demonstrated an increase in receptor antagonists that triggered the development of preeclampsia and pregnancy-induced hypertension.

Prostaglandins

Makrides, Duley, and Olsen (2007) disagreed with the original postulation about prostaglandins found during pregnancy causing changes in the vasculature that leads to preeclampsia. Numerous researchers have compared preeclampsia and normal pregnancies and revealed that in normal pregnancy there is a decreased level of prostacyclin production, whereas thromboxane A2, which is produced by activated platelets, was elevated in those with preeclampsia; however, there was elevation of thromboxane in those with preeclampsia and a low amount of prostacyclin and prostaglandin E2 leading to constriction of the vessels and sensitivity that released angiotensin II. Mignini et al. (2005) and Wallenburg, Dekker, Makovitz, and Rotmans (1991) reported that prevention of hypertension in recurrent pregnancy to maintain angiotensin II should include administration of 81mg aspirin daily. This dosage will decrease the development of thromboxane A2, prostacyclin, and prostaglandin E2. According to Topal et al. (2010), these observations indicated that vessel reactivity may trigger imbalanced hormonal production. Preeclampsia can result from adjustments in a patient's medications.

Although progesterone proved to be a contributing factor to preeclampsia, a progesterone increase during pregnancy is used to maintain pregnancy. Meher and Duley (2009) studied the effects of progesterone during pregnancy with the risk of developing preeclampsia. They discovered that there were not enough reliable data to draw a conclusion. Although progesterone is still an important factor in maintaining pregnancy, its effects and benefits for preventing preeclampsia and its complications still have not been reported.

Vascular Endothelial Growth Factor (VEGF)

VEGF is a cell-producing protein that enhances the supply of oxygen to tissues for growth development. VEGF was seen and documented in placentas after birth. Normally there is a high serum level of VEGF during the first two trimesters at the same time as trophoblast and uterine vascular development in many pregnancies (Bills et al., 2009). Inactive serum VEGF levels in women with preeclampsia indicated a lack of placental growth factor (PIGF), which may be involved in the increased vascular permeability of preeclampsia (Amburgey, Chapman, May, Bernstein, & Cipolla, 2010; Nwosu & Omabe, 2010).

The National Institute of Child Health (2005) stated that decreased blood levels of VEGF in women with preeclampsia increased uteroplacental vessel resistance. It is known that the VEGF physiological response salvages normal blood flow to the placenta. Those with lower levels of VEGF developed preeclampsia, though it also plays an important role in the upkeep of blood vessels. Mignini et al. (2005) described that 50% of women with preeclampsia had antibodies against endothelial cells, whereas 15% were found among normotensive women.

Genetic and Immunological Factors

Dissanayake (2004) studied the multifactorial inheritance of preeclampsia. There was an association between a particular antigen (human leukocyte antigen-DR4) that is seen in women with preeclampsia and those with other diseases like diabetes and hypertension have a genetic predisposition to preeclampsia. Skjaerven et al. (2005) also described inherited genes as part of preeclampsia development. Biggar, Poulsen, Ng, Melbye, and Boyd (2010) described the dysfunction of the immune system between mother and infant that triggered preeclampsia/eclampsia. The sharing of human leukocyte antigen types between the fetus and mother create immune differences. These limitations predispose the mother to a greater risk of preeclampsia. Bonney (2007) wrote that preeclampsia is a result of maternal immunity loss. The successful completion of pregnancy is dependent on the health of the mother's immune system and its ability to carry the pregnancy to full term. Biggar et al. (2010) concluded that the maladaptation of the immune system between mother and infant was found to trigger preeclampsia and eclampsia.

Inflammatory Factors

Dragun and Haase-Fielitz (2009) proposed that the dysfunction of endothelial cells was associated with preeclampsia. This dysfunction was as a result of physiological inflammatory processes in pregnancy. According to Luppi and DeLoia (2006), the leukocyte in the maternal bloodstream triggers cytokines and interleukins that cause oxidation stress related to preeclampsia. There are free radicals such as vitamins E, C, and beta-carotene that later may cause injury to the endothelial cells that balance prostaglandins and nitric oxide in preeclampsia. Huria, Gupta, Kumar, and Sharma (2010) observed the effects of oxidative stress in preeclampsia and the advantages of using antioxidants as a preventive strategy for preeclampsia because antioxidants decrease the level of injured free radicals in the blood (LaMarca et al. 2008; Rani et al., 2010; Vitoratos, Economou, Iavazzo, Panoulis, & Creatsas, 2010). A study by F. Khan (2010) compared demographics and characteristics of normal and preeclamptic pregnant women with serum inflammatory-marker concentrations. There was an association between inflammatory markers of normal pregnancy and women with preeclampsia, further suggesting that a high correlation with inflammatory markers might be an important step in understanding the pathophysiology of preeclampsia.

The Role of Homocysteine

Mignini et al. (2005) documented an increased level of serum homocysteine in normal pregnancy that can lead to preeclampsia.

However, there is a discrepancy in the role of homocysteine in preeclampsia. Kulkarni et al. (2010) described the uncertainty of the association between a higher level of homocysteine and preeclampsia. If a higher level of serum homocysteine is a marker of preeclampsia, then it should be used as a screening tool for early detection. Many quantitative studies demonstrated a cause-and-effect relationship, such that hyperhomocysteine, genetic polymorphisms, folate, and vitamin B12 in pregnancy lead to preeclampsia. A potential benefit of vitamin supplements is in controlling the level of serum homocysteine in pregnancy. In developing countries, many studies have shown relationships between preeclampsia and high levels of homocysteine (Sanchez et al., 2001).

Placenta

A pathological examination compared early normal-delivery placentas and the late onset of preeclampsia. These studies indicated differences between late preeclampsia and normal-term placentas leading to various stages of toxemia (Van der Merwe, Hall, Wright, Schubert, & Grove, 2010). Lindgren, Cederholm, Haglund, and Axelsson (2010) described that the risks of the first—or second-trimester period procedures such as chorionic villus sampling and amniocentesis could cause complications of maternal hypertension and preeclampsia. In another study, Audibert et al. (2010) found that the use of serum markers and uterine artery Doppler in first-time pregnant women (nulliparous) might provide an accurate early screening for preeclampsia. Savvidou, Akolekar, Zaragoza, Poon, and Nicolaides (2009) compared urinary PlGF concentration from 11 weeks to 13 weeks of gestation in women with preeclampsia and normal pregnancies. They concluded that development of preeclampsia was not preceded by altered urinary PlGF concentration in the first trimester of pregnancy. Investigations revealed an association between endothelial dysfunction and blood flow to and from the placenta and preeclampsia. The authors concluded that preexisting endothelial conditions could reduce the placental supply and contribute to the development of preeclampsia. This contradicts all previous studies regarding preeclampsia and its association with the placenta.

Roberts and Gammill (2005) described preeclampsia as a two-stage disease. The first limited blood flow to the placenta, as predicted by previous researchers to be the cause of preeclampsia. The second uncovered death of the umbilical cord wall and a concentration of lipid-laden foam cells with oxidized low-density lipoproteins like the atherosclerotic lesions in preeclampsia (Kim et al., 2007). Levine et al. (2004) confirmed the hypotheses of other researchers that the etiology of preeclampsia was from placental factors in the maternal blood that triggered disorders in endothelial cells, causing proteinuria and elevated blood pressure. This resulted in the elevation of levels of soluble fat-mobilizing substances, possibly preceding preeclampsia.

Risks for Preeclampsia

Powers et al. (2008) described elevated fibronectin in women with preeclampsia and its association with an increased risk of preterm birth. In a study by Craici, Wagner, and Garovic (2008), the authors indicated that about 10% of pregnancies affected by preeclampsia were at risk for future cardiovascular disease. Other metabolic abnormalities cited in a study were obesity and lipid abnormalities (De Ferranti et al., 2004).

Asthma is also associated with preeclampsia because of increased airway hyper-responsiveness found in women, according to a cohort study conducted by Siddiqui et al. (2008). Savvidou et al. (2009) compared PIGF concentration during an 11- to 13-week gestation period in women with preeclampsia and normotensive pregnancy. They determined that the development of preeclampsia was not preceded by altered PIGF concentrations in the first trimester of pregnancy, as previous studies portrayed. According to Thadhani and Solomon (2008), the risk of preeclampsia associated with nulliparity, extremes of maternal age, obesity, and preexisting diabetes or hypertension, however, remained uncertain. Current documentation has shown other factors—angiogenesis rennin and insulin—involved in the development of preeclampsia (Thadhani & Solomon, 2008). Despite several attempts to implement various treatments, there has not been an effective way to prevent or treat preeclampsia except delivery of the baby.

Guidelines for Preeclampsia

Due to this devastating disease, many researchers developed guidelines for practitioners to follow, such as the Preeclampsia Community Guideline (Milne et al., 2005). They reviewed the evidence and requirements for women suspected of having preeclampsia. The National Institute for Health and Clinical Excellence, developed by Nicolaides et al. (2006), also provided early guidance for healthcare providers to manage preeclampsia and other hypertensive disorders during pregnancy to promote health in mother and baby. According to Smith et al. (2002), these international scientists described the combination of recent technologies and the results of data collected to detect preeclampsia in early pregnancy. The metabolites showed the risk of preeclampsia by using the screening-for-pregnancy-endpoints method, providing easy, affordable, and accessible blood tests to predict and prevent preeclampsia and its complications. These guidelines were never practically implemented and are not presently used as a gold standard in practice. Bridges, Womble, Wallace, and McCartney (2003) found the central pressure in the veins of preeclamptic women did not correlate with the pulmonary-artery wedge pressure of a normal pregnancy. Bridges et al. recommended monitoring pregnancy at 20 weeks of gestation. The importance of protocol in follow-up assessments, and recognizing early treatment of preeclampsia cannot be overemphasized.

Clinical Presentations of Other Diseases With Preeclampsia

According to Bellamy, Casas, Hingorani, and Williams (2007), most preeclamptic women have clinical findings of cardiovascular disease, though it differs in severity and duration. Unrecognized chronic diseases may present differently, and treatment of these underlying conditions may affect some clinical manifestations. Preeclampsia and eclampsia can cause pathological changes in normal cardiovascular function. The manifestation of these changes is hypertension due to cardiac afterload, whereas the cardiac preload will cause hypovolemia and increased activities of endothelia in pregnancy. The pathophysiology of preeclampsia is recognized during the development of chorionic villi in pregnancy. It was documented that these excessive chorionic villi in maternal serum predispose pregnant women to hypertension, and if untreated may lead to preeclampsia (Karumanchi, Maynard, Sukhatme, Stillman, & Epstein, 2005).

Detection and Theory of the Processes of Change

The HBM is a scaffold that scrutinizes participation in health behaviors among individuals and a criterion of health-education management (Rosenstock et al., 1988). HBM is based on the concept that knowledge, attitude, belief, and perception are barriers to the decision-making ability of an individual. In the same way, health education encourages and compares the positive and negative aspects of the disease outcome and the willingness to change health beliefs.

Researchers work to expand knowledge of numerous disease findings, and how to better understand why pregnant women will want to know more about preeclampsia and needs for health promotion through public health, communities, and individuals. Adults indulge in self-efficacy to perform health-related interventions after health-education awareness and knowledge of the threats are understood (Rosenstock et al., 1988).

The HBM can bring an understanding and prediction of behavior to help people practice healthy behaviors. Education and knowledge of causal processes of preeclampsia will highly motivate behavior and bring about success. Only then can people be persuaded to use health services for designated problems (Rosenstock, 2005, p. 94). HBM, as documented by various researchers, can be used to investigate numerous health behaviors in populations that are diverse (Denison, 1996). According to Bandura (1989), researchers believe that success in health beliefs and behaviors are the perceptions of individuals about threatened poor health, realized through education and knowledge of disease. Improved treatment remains a critical public health challenge; multifaceted interventions are found to be most effective (Grol, 2001). These require a combination of different steps to bring about motivational changes such as promoting education and counseling in patients, involving patients in their care, bringing accessibility of care to patient, tips to remember in a calendar, and incentives (Grol, 2001).

Education and Counseling in Prevention

Okafor and Ezegwui (2010) indicated that education and counseling for women may help women plan pregnancies in cases where risk factors are obvious. However, Munger et al. (2007) agreed with Grol (2001) on the use of effective strategies, like promoting teaching and counseling in patients about the process of preeclampsia, involving patients in their care, bringing accessible care to patients, tips to remember in a calendar, and incentives to produced a desirable outcome. Despite these different treatments producing successes, there were numerous pitfalls. It was not easy to invent ways that worked for every patient.

Studies on Population

Preeclampsia has been described as being caused by a triad of proteinuria, hypertension, and edema. Population studies around the world have shown that preeclampsia and eclampsia rank among the most common complications of pregnancy, resulting in high morbidity, especially in developing countries. Rawashdeh (2010) described preeclampsia as a disease with multisystem disorders in obstetrics and a most virulent cause of both morbidity and mortality.

K. Khan et al. (2006) maintained that the leading cause of maternal deaths in Latin American and Caribbean countries are preeclampsia and pregnancy-induced hypertension disorders. They assessed the causes as a complex set of mechanisms associated with a variety of fetal and maternal risk factors that originated from familial genes, maternal behavior, or environmental disposition.

Overall, the development of preeclampsia has been attributed to different genetic, nongenetic, and immunological factors. Chikosi, Moodley, Pegoraro, Lanning, and Rom (1999) indicated that gene 5, 10-methylenelehahydrofolate reductase (MTHFR), was associated with the enzyme homocysteine, increasing the risk of preeclampsia in Black South African women, and documented that most maternal mortality in South African women was caused by preeclampsia. Although MTHFR could not be directly linked to preeclampsia in South African women, there was a genetic factor that influenced women who would later contract this disease (Hira, Pegoraro, Rom, & Moodley, 2003). A similar study conducted by Pérez-Mutul, González-Herrera, Sosa-Cabrera, and Martínez-Olivares (2004) in women of southeast Mexico suggested no association between MTHFR and preeclampsia.

The protein tyrosine kinase increased the risk of preeclampsia and the level of soluble fat-mobilizing substance in the placenta of South African women. Yeo, Wells, Kieffer, and Nolan (2007) estimated its incidence among Hispanic women and found that this grouping had a lower risk of developing preeclampsia or pregnancy-induced hypertension compared to other ethnic groups in the delivery book. High levels of cotinine also indicted decreased risk for preeclampsia in African American women. Earlier studies maintained that women who smoked would harm the growing fetus. A study by Janakiraman, Gantz, Maynard, and El-Mohandes (2009) tested the theory that reduced risk of preeclampsia was due to nicotine in the serum after smoking and found no support for it.

López-Pulles et al. (2010) proposed that immunogenetic factors caused the development of preeclampsia in Ecuadorian women. Their findings, however, were inconclusive. Five percent of Sri Lankan women are affected by preeclampsia during pregnancy due to genetic and environmental factors. Researchers documented Sinhalese women with great morbidity in relation to preeclampsia. They highlighted common features between the allele and haplotype of Sri Lankan women that occurred more than in Caucasians (Dissanayake, 2004). Patrick, Powers, Daftary, Ness, and Roberts (2004) stated that plasma homocysteine in Black women may have caused an increased risk of preeclampsia. These authors compared plasma homocysteine, folic acid, and B12, according to race. Their findings were inconclusive.

Finn (2005) investigated Hispanic women who developed preeclampsia in their late gestation period and found their preeclampsia was less severe than in other ethnicities. There was no significant difference due to genetic factors. The low-dose effect of aspirin in preeclamptic nulliparous women and its manifestations were thoroughly reviewed by Ruano, Fontes, and Zugaib (2005).

Semenovskaya and Erogul (2010) described preeclampsia as an anomaly of the endothelial vessels that occurred at 20 weeks of gestation or 4 to 6 weeks after delivery and resulted in stillbirth and neonatal death. HIV/AIDS and preeclampsia are fatal diseases in developing countries, according to Hall (2007). Hall researched whether HIV lowered the rate of preeclampsia. HIV/AIDS and preeclampsia had high rates in South Africa and caused morbidity and mortality. Because this study is ongoing, it will take 3 years to produce a result.

Studies from other cultures are being conducted. For example, Chinese herbal medicines are used in the treatment of preeclampsia. Chinese-medicine researchers suggested that the flow of blood supply going to the placenta provided the fetus with the required nutrition to protect the baby from preeclampsia. They urged encouraging vasodilatation, increased blood flow, and decreased platelet aggregation (Li et al., 2009). Researchers found that Black women in Dallas had more highly elevated blood pressure and decreased folic acid with amino acid than did White women. The authors investigated the preexisting risk factors for preeclampsia and discovered that homocysteine was elevated in women with preeclampsia. These factors were associated with how folic acid appeared in their diet (Dallas Researchers, 2004; Ingec, Borekci, & Kadanali, 2005). Mulla, Gonzalez-Sanchez, and Nuwayhid (2007) calculated preeclampsia hospital-discharge rates in Florida. They concluded that preeclampsia was a cause of prolonged length of stay in the hospital due to the disease.

Studies in Nigeria

Approximately one third of the maternal deaths in Nigeria are due to the complication of pregnancy, toxemia, known as preeclampsia (Abubakar et al., 2009). Chigbu, Okezie, and Odugu (2009) studied women in their second pregnancies and determined the significance of preeclampsia between women who had moved from original partners and women who remained with the same partner, in all parts of southern Nigeria. The incidence of preeclampsia increased in women who had paternal changes for subsequent pregnancy and the duration of sexual cohabitation among those with changed partners for conception at interpregnancy intervals. At 24-weeks gestation there was no significant difference among women who changed partners in serum free radicals and decreased amounts of antioxidant vitamins. To prevent preeclampsia, calcium and magnesium supplements were given to Nigerian women with preeclampsia and eclampsia. The results indicted reduction of extracellular calcium and magnesium among these women corresponding with preeclampsia (Idogun, Imarengiaye, & Momoh, 2007).

A prospective cohort study by Chigbu et al. (2009) revealed that hypertensive Nigerian women have a higher risk for preeclampsia in the middle trimester of pregnancy. High blood pressure can influence fetal brain development and be a factor in preexisting chronic hypertension. Uboh et al. (2008) suggested that an increase in malonyldialdehyde and a decrease in antioxidant vitamins were the main causes for preeclampsia in Nigerian women. Pregnancy-induced hypertension was documented as one of the leading complications among adolescents. This elevated blood pressure, if unrecognized, may lead to preeclampsia and later to eclampsia. The adverse results of untreated eclampsia are kidney and retinal problems, chronic hypertension, congestive heart failure, stroke, or death.

Igberase and Ebeigbe (2006) and Olopade and Lawoyin (2008) conducted studies in Nigeria and found that of pregnant women who were 15 years old and younger, 40% had preeclampsia. In the United States the range of preeclampsia is 2-6% in first-time pregnancies, whereas, in developing countries, that range is reported to be 4-18%. In Nigeria it was documented that 75% cases of preeclampsia were mild and 25% severe; 10% occur in pregnancies of less than 34 weeks' gestation. The estimation is that eclampsia occurs in 1 in 200 cases of preeclampsia without early detection or prompt administration of magnesium sulfate (Igberase & Ebeigbe, 2006; Olopade & Lawoyin, 2008).

Okafor and Ezegwui (2010) studied seasonal variations in cesarean-section deliveries. Patients with a history of preeclampsia/eclampsia were counseled to plan pregnancies in advance to reduce the morbidity and mortality associated with seasonally induced preeclampsia. Shaarawy et al. (2005) also investigated the variation in seasons in the presentation of preeclampsia and caesarean-section deliveries in the tropical rainforest. They found no significance. An investigation of hospital records from July 1998 to June 2006 yielded maternal-mortality risk factors related to anesthesia during caesarean in preeclamptic women. Okafor, Efetie, Igwe, and Okezie (2009) found that the cause of fetal demise in developing countries was preeclampsia/eclampsia, even with the availability of obstetric care. The conclusion of their study was that early treatment during preeclampsia maintains placental blood supply in cases where anesthesia is required, thereby reducing perinatal mortality (Okafor et al., 2009).

Methods

Quantitative Research

Many studies included in the literature review were both quantitative and qualitative and provided a profusion of information about Nigerian women's risk factors, causes, and perceptions of preeclampsia. The key element of this study was to investigate the attitude and perception of preeclampsia among first-generation Nigerian women living in the United States. It is necessary to adapt a method that will demonstrate the requirement of study participants to describe their experiences, thoughts, and behaviors. Creswell (2003) defined methods as processes and steps used in accumulating and analyzing data. Carter and Little (2007) described the key elements of research methods such as the sampling, collecting data, management of data, analysis of data, and reporting of data.

The most important characteristic of quantitative research is the use of numeric data (Ulin et al., 2005). The focus of quantitative research is collecting information through questionnaires or surveys that are used to measure feelings and other factors numerically. Various relationships of variables can be used to measure statistical data (Creswell, 2003). The selection of quantitative research in this study is therefore appropriate to address the problem in this study.

Similar studies have taken advantage of quantitative research methods to describe Nigerian women with preeclampsia. Hofmeyr et al. (2010) used a quantitative research method to ascertain the use calcium supplements to minimize the debilitating and fatal outcomes of preeclampsia. Also, Abubakar et al. (2009) compared Hausa, Fulani, and Kanuri preeclamptic women in northern Nigeria using a quantitative method and found elevated values of triglyceride, serum cholesterol, pathological edema, increase in blood pressure, and higher values of urine protein among the Hausa and the Kanuri women than among Fulani preeclamptic women. This research pointed to the likelihood that Fulani women would progress to eclampsia more than members of the other two tribes.

Quantitative methods will facilitate the investigation of attitudes and perceptions of preeclampsia among first-generation Nigerian women living in United States. There are traditional approaches to quantitative research using survey and experimental methods. A quantitative research design is chosen in contrast to a qualitative research design because the researcher used postpositivist steps to develop variables and hypotheses (Creswell, 2003).

There are two types of quantitative methodologies in descriptive and experimental research. Descriptive research does not determine cause-effect relationships that indicate patterns among the variables. Collecting data and testing research questions about concerns are part of descriptive research and findings are reported accordingly. Experimental research describes cause and effect relationships, and shows comparisons with possible causes. According to Creswell (2002), the independent variable as a cause and the dependent variable as an effect make the research salient. A survey approach to an inquiry research methodology will be restricted to participants' experiences, with the aim of understanding those experiences; understanding is the goal of healthcare research (Creswell, 2007, p. 62). Even though other research approaches are reviewed, survey inquiry offers the most appropriate method for exploring attitudes and perceptions about preeclampsia among first-generation Nigerian women.

Data collection, data analysis, and interpretation of data are commonly used in quantitative research. It also uses statistics to analyze the specific ways to solve problems (Soemarno, 2007), whereas qualitative research uses texts, images, and pictures as the base (Creswell, 2003). Surveys, sampling, and data collection are required to determine numerical value and have the ability to be counted (Creswell, 2003). Quantitative researchers use many methodologies to determine the way different of people act, think, and feel.

Instrumentation

The most important aspect of quantitative research is to determine the appropriate method of data collection and instruments to measure the variables. The different methods are experiment and survey. In the experimental method, participants are assigned randomly to treatment or control groups. In quasi-experiment, researchers work with a nonrandomized design. In contrast, surveys use no treatment or control groups; they use questionnaires for larger populations (Creswell, 2003).

Types of Methods That Could Have Been Used

As described above, the subject of preeclampsia has been studied by many authors (Igberase & Ebeigbe, 2006: Janakiraman et al., 2009; LaMarca et al., 2008; Nicolaides et al., 2006; Okafor & Ezegwui, 2010; Olopade & Lawoyin, 2008) who used different methods, from qualitative (case-studies or individual interviews) to quantitative (surveys or clinical experiments with interventions); others used mixed methods (both focus groups and surveys), though few researchers used this approach. Mixed methods are a combination of quantitative and qualitative design in a single study and are popular in health-science research, whereas surveys are commonly used in quantitative inquiry.

Summary

Preeclampsia has been studied, with many researchers attempting to predict causes, risk factors, and management. There is a need to educate women to expand their understanding of causes and risk factors, to enhance prompt and early recognition of preeclampsia. The aim is to reduce the severity of the debilitation of the disease and its associated consequences. The lack of standard guidelines to diagnose preeclampsia and promote health for women continues.

The goal of Chapter 2 was to review the existing documentation on risk factors, causes, and management of preeclampsia. Chapter 2 also described studies on attitudes, perceptions, and experiences of various ethnic groups worldwide. Chapter 3 will discuss the methodology, design, sample and study setting, collection of data, analysis, and ethical issues related to this study.

CHAPTER 3

Research Method

This chapter presents the research design, sample, instruments, research questions, selection of participants, collection of data, data analysis, and ethical considerations. The quantitative study assessed the knowledge, attitudes, and perceptions of preeclampsia among first-generation Nigerian women with a history of preeclampsia living in the United States from their perspective, as well as reviewed their understanding of early recognition of preeclampsia. The study was designed to advance the body of knowledge regarding preeclampsia in first-generation Nigerian women diagnosed or previously diagnosed, living in the United States. This study addressed the gap in the literature exploring preeclampsia from the perspective of first-generation Nigerian women living in the United States who have been affected by preeclampsia. This study took place while assessing the present and potential risks of women with a history of the disease. The findings may increase the body of knowledge on the understanding of various risk factors, different theories, and the study of preeclampsia in different cultures and ethnic groups. The study will reinforce early recognition and treatment by obstetricians.

Research Design

A cross-sectional survey was administered to first-generation Nigerian women with a history of preeclampsia living in the United States. The survey contained mainly quantitative questions addressing various aspects of knowledge, attitudes, and perceptions of preeclampsia and important factors including demographic characteristics and other respondent characteristics.

Participants of the Study

The population targeted was first-generation Nigerian women with a history of preeclampsia or eclampsia residing in the Queens, Brooklyn, Bronx, and Long Island areas of New York. This study participants included women who are pregnant or have been pregnant and were diagnosed with preeclampsia at 20 weeks of gestation and had a baby or who experienced preeclampsia in past pregnancies. Approximately 180 first-generation Nigerian women ($N = 180$) were needed as participants to achieve a significant result, if it existed. The sampling was purposeful with 25%, $n = 45$, representing each area of New York (specifically Queens, Brooklyn, Bronx, and Long Island). The strategy of this approach was initiated for two reasons: the target population was the audience of interest and was able to provide the needed information. The size was determined using Cohen's *d* (Cohen, 1988) calculation to obtain the effect size. Cohen (1988) used three imaginary values as standard effect sizes: .20 is a "small effect," .50 is a "medium effect," .80 is a "large effect," but small and medium effect sizes are commonly used in social and behavioral research. The medium size was the target at the *alpha* = .05 significance level for a two-tailed test with a power of 0.80 for this study.

Recruitment of study participants was conducted through advertisements posted in Nigerian churches and African markets and through individual distribution of flyers. Participants were solicited through many sources such as braiding salons, Nigerian churches, grocery stores, physicians' offices, universities, community centers, and word-of-mouth. The criteria for the purposive sample selection represent only a small sample of the target population, allowing for an easy way of seeking a particular group of people (Trochim, 2006).

Purposive sampling technique was the main method to recruit first-generation Nigerian women living in the United States. Purposive sampling is proper for cases in which the researcher's aim is to get the opinions of the target group and there is a need to reach a targeted group quickly when proportionality is not the major concern (Trochim, 2006). Thus, the selection was a nonprobability purposive sample of women who met the criteria of the study (Ulin et al., 2005).

Inclusion and Exclusion Criteria

The criteria for inclusion are first-generation Nigerian women living in the New York area who are pregnant and diagnosed with preeclampsia or previously pregnant and had an episode of preeclampsia and who are 18 years or older. Exclusive criteria was nonfirst-generation Nigerian women, women from other African countries, reported cases not associated with preeclampsia, self-reported cases of preeclampsia with no clinical documentation sought to confirm diagnosis of this illness, and cases of high blood pressure in pregnancy that could be reported as preeclampsia.

Instrumentation

The survey instruments were compiled after reviewing the literature, getting expert opinion, receiving input from maternal-health and health-education specialists, and based on the personal experience of the researcher in such studies. The survey instrument assessing knowledge, attitudes, and perceptions of preeclampsia was a version of a survey developed by East, Conway, Pollack, Frawley, and Brennecke (2011). The questionnaire from East et al. assessed knowledge, attitudes, and perceptions of preeclampsia and participants' experience prior to hospitalization. Participants were asked to recall their perceptions of their experiences of preeclampsia symptoms, prenatal visits to a physician's office, and hospitalization. Responses for the items addressing knowledge, attitudes, and perceptions of preeclampsia were a mix of dichotomous (yes/no), categorical, continuous, and ordinal (recorded on a 5-point Likert-type scale: *strongly disagree, disagree, neutral, agree, strongly agree*) variables. This survey was tested for validity and reliability in East et al.'s study. The internal consistency and reliability were validated based on alpha/correlation/ factor analysis (East et al., 2011). East and colleagues granted permission to use this tool for this research. No changes were made to the original instrument assessing knowledge, attitudes, and perceptions of preeclampsia. There was an additional questionnaire included addressing participant socioeconomic and demographic data pertinent to the research question (Wilson, 2009). The participant-demographic portion was comprised of personal data and other necessary variables such as age, gravidity, parity, cultural beliefs, technology, education, acculturation, socioeconomic status, access to health care, whether they have children, any history of preeclampsia or hypertension, and gestational age. Responses for the items addressing cultural beliefs, education, socioeconomic status, acculturation, and technology were a mix of dichotomous (yes/no), categorical, continuous, and ordinal (recorded on a 5-point Likert-type scale: *strongly disagree, disagree, neutral, agree, strongly agree*) variables.

Research Questions and Hypotheses

Research Question 1: Is there a relationship between demographic characteristics, cultural beliefs, socioeconomic status, acculturation, and access to health care and knowledge of preeclampsia among first-generation Nigerian women with a history of preeclampsia living in the United States?

*H*a: Demographic characteristics, cultural beliefs, socioeconomic status, acculturation, and access to health care will be significantly related to knowledge of preeclampsia among first-generation Nigerian women with a history of preeclampsia living in the United States.

*H*0: There is no relationship between demographic characteristics, cultural beliefs, socioeconomic status, acculturation, and access to health care and knowledge of preeclampsia among first-generation Nigerian women with a history of preeclampsia living in the United States.

Research Question 2: Is there a relationship between demographic characteristics, cultural beliefs, socioeconomic status, acculturation, and access to health care and attitudes of preeclampsia among first-generation Nigerian women with a history of preeclampsia living in the United States?

*H*a: Demographic characteristics, cultural beliefs, socioeconomic status, acculturation, and access to health care will be significantly related to attitudes of preeclampsia among first-generation Nigerian women with a history of preeclampsia living in the United States.

*H*0: There is no relationship between demographic characteristics, cultural beliefs, socioeconomic status, acculturation, and access to health care and attitudes of preeclampsia among first-generation Nigerian women with a history of preeclampsia living in the United States.

Research Question 3: Is there a relationship between demographic characteristics, cultural beliefs, socioeconomic status, acculturation, and access to health care and perceptions of preeclampsia among first-generation Nigerian women with a history of preeclampsia living in the United States?

*H*a: Demographic characteristics, cultural beliefs, socioeconomic status, acculturation, and access to health care will be significantly related to perceptions of preeclampsia among first-generation Nigerian women with a history of preeclampsia living in the United States.

*H*0: There is no relationship between demographic characteristics, cultural beliefs, socioeconomic status, acculturation, and access to health care and perceptions of preeclampsia among first-generation Nigerian women with a history of preeclampsia living in the United States.

Data Collection Procedures

The survey was created online and participants completed the survey online via SurveyMonkey. The questionnaire was documented as an online SurveyMonkey questionnaire on the webpage. The potential participants accessed a link on the flyer. Buffering measures were instituted to prevent withdrawal and incomplete responses to the survey, creating a strict rule and environment for the participants as a guideline, such as a 3-week deadline for potential participants to return the survey, e-mail reminders, and closing the survey after another week. These measures served to protect the well-being and rights of participants, informed consent, and ensuring that participants who wished to withdraw were not penalized. Participants responded to flyers and notices regarding participation in the study by accessing the link on the flyers.

The researcher recorded the web address on the flyers; interested participants who accessed the website implied consent through the explanation of the study. Participants were given many opportunities to withdraw from the study, including during the initial contact with the researcher. Participants filled out and submitted the survey questionnaire online via the SurveyMonkey website. Participants who were unable or unwilling to complete the survey were excluded from the study. Potential study participants were given 3 weeks to complete the survey and subsequently were excluded from the study. If study participants contacted the researcher prior to the end of the data collection phase, they could still be included in the study. Data were checked for completeness and consistency by a data "consistency checks" procedure during the initial contact with participants through the collection of the data online.

Data Analysis

After collecting the data using SurveyMonkey, they were exported and analyzed with SPSS 17.0 to test the hypothesis that respondent characteristics were related to knowledge, attitudes, and perceptions of preeclampsia. The dependent and independent variables were binary and ordinal logistic regressions using significance testing. Logistic regression allowed the prediction of the outcome and determined a relationship between the dependent variable and independent variables. Logistic regression also demonstrated understanding of a relationship within the variables and resolved inconsistencies in relation to the dependent variable. Logistic regression generated a coefficients formula to predict a *logit transformation*. Logistic regression is used more with health-related studies. All knowledge, attitude, and perception variables were ordinal (responses ranging from *strongly disagree* to *strongly agree*). The respondent characteristics variables were a mix of continuous, ordinal, and binary variables. The logistic regression approach chosen determined the relationship of many variables. In regression analysis, the odds ratios and confidence intervals were illustrated. If the confidence intervals (CIs) did not include 1.0, then results are significant at $p < 005$. For example, a CI of 1.2-2-4 means that it is significant at $p < 05$. Logistic and ordinal logistic regressio were reported along with *p*-values, determining if a relationship was statistically significant at $p < . 05$.

Variables involved follow:

- 14 dependent variables

    - Knowledge of preeclampsia PE: experiences3a, experiences4a, experiences4c, experiences4d, experiences8a

        i. Experiences3a: During my pregnancy but before I was diagnosed with preeclampsia, I knew about preeclampsia. (1 = *a lot*, 2 = *a little*, 3 = *very little*, 4 = *not at all*, 5 = *undecided*)

        ii. Expeerinces4a: When I was diagnosed with preeclampsia, I thought it could not happen to me. (1 = *strongly agree*, 2 = *agree*, 3 = *disagree*, 4 = *strongly disagree*, 5 = *undecided*)

        iii. Experiences4c: When I was diagnosed with preeclampsia, I thought it was not serious or life threatening. (1 = *strongly agree*, 2 = *agree*, 3 = *disagree*, 4 = *strongly disagree*, 5 = *undecided*)

        iv. Experiences4d: When I was diagnosed with preeclampsia, I was frightened. (1 = *strongly agree*, 2 = *agree*, 3 = *disagree*, 4 = *strongly disagree*, 5 = *undecided*)

v. Experiences8a: In the weeks, months, or years since my preeclampsia experience, I had professional counseling to talk about my experience. (Yes/No)

- Attitude of preeclampsia: experiences5a, experiences5e, experiences5f, experiences9a, experiences9b

    i. Experiences5a: As the preeclampsia continued or become more severe, I felt that I had lost control of my destiny. (1 = *strongly agree*, 2 = *agree*, 3 = *disagree*, 4 = *strongly disagree*, 5 = *undecided*)

    ii. Experiences5e: As the preeclampsia continued or become more severe, I felt that no one around me had been through the same experience as I had. (1 = *strongly agree*, 2 = *agree*, 3 = *disagree*, 4 = *strongly disagree*, 5 = *undecided*)

    iii. Experiences5f: As the preeclampsia continued or become more severe, I did not realize how sick I really was. (1 = *strongly agree*, 2 = *agree*, 3 = *disagree*, 4 = *strongly disagree*, 5 = *undecided*)

    iv. Experiences9a: My experience with preeclampsia influenced how long it was between the preeclampsia pregnancy and the next pregnancy. (1 = *strongly agree*, 2 = *agree*, 3 = *disagree*, 4 = *strongly disagree*, 5 = *undecided*)

    v. Experiences9b: Having had preeclampsia before influenced my feelings, choices, and care during the next pregnancy with respect to enjoyment of pregnancy. (1 = *strongly agree*, 2 = *agree*, 3 = *disagree*, 4 = *strongly disagree*, 5 = *undecided*)

- Perception of preeclampsia: experiences7a, experiences7b, experiences8b, experiences8k

    i. Experiences7a: I felt that my ability to initially bond with my baby was limited because I was so sick. (1 = *strongly* agree, 2 = *agree*, 3 = *disagree*, 4 = *strongly disagree*, 5 = *undecided*)

ii. Experiences7b: I felt that my ability to initially bond with my baby was limited because my baby was so sick. (1 = *strongly agree*, 2 = *agree*, 3 = *disagree*, 4 = *strongly disagree*, 5 = *undecided*)

iii. Experiences8b: In the weeks, months, or years since my preeclampsia experience, I felt the need to obtain more information about preeclampsia. (Yes/No)

iv. Experiences8k: In the weeks, months or years since my preeclampsia experience, my baby has needed extra healthcare. (1 = *strongly agree*, 2 = *agree*, 3 = *disagree*, 4 = *strongly disagree*, 5 = *undecided*)

- Independent variables

  - Demographics: participants questionnaire_a, participants questionnaire_b, participants questionnaire_c, participants questionnaire_d, participants questionnaire_e (PQ-participants questionnaire)

    i. PQ_a: are you a first-generation Nigeria woman? (Yes/No)
    ii. PQ_b: are you pregnant? (Yes/No)
    iii. PQ_c: Did you have preeclampsia in a previous pregnancy? (Yes/No)
    iv. PQ_d: Are you or were you 18 years or older when you first experienced preeclampsia? (Yes/No)

  - Socioeconomic status: Socioeconomic status_e, Socioeconomic status_f, Socioeconomic status_g, Socioeconomic status_h, Socioeconomic status_i

    i. Sedds_e: What is your employment status? (employed full time, employed part time, unemployed, other)

    ii. Sedds_f: what is your current marital status? (married, single, divorced, widow, separated)

    iii. Sedds_g: Which of the following describes your highest level of educational attainment? (Less than high school, high school or general education development (GED), some college, associate's degree, bachelor's degree, postgraduate degree)

    iv. Sedds_h: Do you collect Women, Infants, and Children (WIC)? (Yes/No)

    v. Sedds_i: Do you currently have health insurance? (Yes/No)

- Acculturation: experiences8g, experiences8h, experiences8i, experiences8m

    i. Experiences8g: In the weeks, months, or years since my preeclampsia experience, I have found that talking or writing about my experience with preeclampsia has helped me. (1 = *strongly agree*, 2 = *agree*, 3 = *disagree*, 4 = *strongly disagree*, 5 = *undecided*)

    ii. Experiences8h: In the weeks, months, or years since my preeclampsia experience, I have had very little confidence in my mothering ability. (1 = *strongly agree*, 2 = *agree*, 3 = *disagree*, 4 = *strongly disagree*, 5 = *undecided*)

    iii. Experiences8i: In the weeks, months or years since my preeclampsia experience, I have had a strong sense of self-worth. (1 = *strongly agree*, 2 = *agree*, 3 = *disagree*, 4 = *strongly disagree*, 5 = *undecided*)

    iv. Experiences8m: In the weeks, months, or years since my preeclampsia experience, I have become aware that there may be a genetic link for preeclampsia; for example, my mother had preeclampsia. (1 = *strongly agree*, 2 = *agree*, 3 = *disagree*, 4 = *strongly disagree*, 5 = *undecided*)

- Access to health care: experiences4e, experiences6a, experiences6c

    i. Experiences4e: When I was diagnosed with preeclampsia, I felt a sense of having let myself down by becoming sick with preeclampsia (1 = *strongly agree*, 2 = *agree*, 3 = *disagree*, 4 = *strongly disagree*, 5 = *undecided*).

    ii. Experiences6a: Did your experience of preeclampsia result in the death of your baby? (Yes/No)

    iii. Experiences6c: Did you feel supported by the hospital staff following your baby's death? (Yes/No). Note that as expe6c was a suquestion of expe6a, not all subjects answered this question. Hence, expe6c was not used as one of the independent variables in the following analysis (see Tables 1, 2, and 3).

Table 1
Variable Table

Q#	Question	Label (from East et al., 2011)	Response option	Data type	Analysis notes
3a	During my pregnancy but before I was diagnosed with PE, I knew about PE:	Life perceptions and knowledge prior to diagnosis of preeclampsia: No knowledge of PE	1 A lot 2 A little 3 Very little 4 Not at all 5 Undecided	Ordinal	Ordinal Logistic Regression
4a	When I was diagnosed with PE, I thought it couldn't happen to me	Following diagnosis with PE: Thought it could not happen to her	1 Strongly agree 2 Agree 3 Disagree 4 Strongly Disagree 5 Undecided	Ordinal	Ordinal Logistic Regression
4c	When I was diagnosed with PE, I thought it was not serious or life threatening	Following diagnosis with PE: Thought it was not serious or life threatening	1 Strongly agree 2 Agree 3 Disagree 4 Strongly Disagree 5 Undecided	Ordinal	Ordinal Logistic Regression
4d	When I was diagnosed with PE, I was frightened	Following diagnosis with PE: Was frightened	1 Strongly agree 2 Agree 3 Disagree 4 Strongly Disagree 5 Undecided	Ordinal	Ordinal Logistic Regression
5a	As the PE continued or became more severe, I felt that I had lost control of my destiny	As the PE continued or became more severe: Felt had lost control of own destiny	1 Strongly agree 2 Agree 3 Disagree 4 Strongly Disagree 5 Undecided	Ordinal	Ordinal Logistic Regression
5e	As the PE continued or became more severe, I felt that no one around me had been through the same experience as I had	As the PE continued or became more severe: Felt that no-one around had been through same experiences	1 Strongly agree 2 Agree 3 Disagree 4 Strongly Disagree 5 Undecided	Ordinal	Ordinal Logistic Regression

Q#	Question	Label (from East et al., 2011)	Response option	Data type	Analysis notes
5f	As the PE continued or became more severe, I did not realize how sick I really was	*NA (not in paper)* As the PE continued or became more severe: Did not realize how sick I was	1 Strongly agree 2 Agree 3 Disagree 4 Strongly Disagree 5 Undecided	Ordinal	Ordinal Logistic Regression
6g	How my preeclampsia affected my early experience with my baby/babies, I felt that my baby might die	How the PE affected early experiences with the baby/babies: Felt that baby might die	1 Strongly agree 2 Agree 3 Disagree 4 Strongly Disagree 5 Undecided	Ordinal	Ordinal Logistic Regression
7a	I felt that my ability to initially bond with my baby was limited because I was too sick	Feelings that her ability to bond with the baby were limited, because: As a mother, she was too sick	1 Strongly agree 2 Agree 3 Disagree 4 Strongly Disagree 5 Undecided	Ordinal	Ordinal Logistic Regression
7b	I felt that my ability to initially bond with my baby was limited because my baby was too sick	Feelings that her ability to bond with the baby were limited, because: The baby was too sick	1 Strongly agree 2 Agree 3 Disagree 4 Strongly Disagree 5 Undecided	Ordinal	Ordinal Logistic Regression
8a	In the weeks, months or years since my PE experience . . . I have had professional counseling to talk about my experience	In the weeks, months, or years since the PE experience: Had professional counseling to talk about the experience	1 No 2 Yes	Binary	Logistic Regression
8b	In the weeks, months or years since my PE experience . . . I felt the need to obtain more information about PE	In the weeks, months, or years since the PE experience: Felt the need to obtain more information about PE	1 No 2 Yes	Binary	Logistic Regression

Q#	Question	Label (from East et al., 2011)	Response option	Data type	Analysis notes
8h	In the weeks, months or years since my PE experience . . . I have had very little confidence in my mothering ability	In the weeks, months, or years since the PE experience: Have had very little confidence in mothering ability	1 Strongly agree 2 Agree 3 Disagree 4 Strongly Disagree 5 Undecided	Ordinal	Ordinal Logistic Regression
8k	In the weeks, months or years since my PE experience . . . My baby has needed extra healthcare	In the weeks, months, or years since the PE experience: Consider the baby has needed extra healthcare	1 Strongly agree 2 Agree 3 Disagree 4 Strongly Disagree 5 Undecided	Ordinal	Ordinal Logistic Regression
8i	In the weeks, months or years since my PE experience . . . I have felt increased anxiety toward future pregnancies	How women considered their experience of PE affected later pregnancies: Felt increased anxiety toward future pregnancies	1 Strongly agree 2 Agree 3 Disagree 4 Strongly Disagree 5 Undecided	Ordinal	Ordinal Logistic Regression
9a	We are interested in how your experience of PE affected later pregnancies. My experience with PE influenced how long it was between the PE pregnancy and the next pregnancy (you may still be contemplating the next pregnancy)	How women considered their experience of PE affected later pregnancies: PE experience influenced interval to next pregnancy	1 Strongly agree 2 Agree 3 Disagree 4 Strongly Disagree 5 Undecided	Ordinal	Ordinal Logistic Regression

Q#	Question	Label (from East et al., 2011)	Response option	Data type	Analysis notes
9b	Having had PE before influenced my feelings, choices, and care during the next pregnancy with respect to enjoyment of the pregnancy	How women considered their experience of PE affected later pregnancies: Enjoyment of the pregnancy	1 Strongly agree 2 Agree 3 Disagree 4 Strongly Disagree 5 Undecided	Ordinal	Ordinal Logistic Regression
A	Are you first-generation Nigeria woman?	Participant Questionnaire	1. Yes 2. No	Binary	Logistic Regression
B	Are you pregnant?	Participant Questionnaire	1. Yes 2. No	Binary	Logistic Regression
C	Do you have any history of preeclampsia?	Participant Questionnaire	1. Yes 2. No	Binary	Logistic Regression
D	What is your current marital status?	Participant Questionnaire	1. Married 2. Single 3. Divorced 4. Widow 5. Separated	Ordinal	Ordinal Logistic Regression
E	Which of the following describes your highest level of education attainment	Participant Questionnaire	1. Less than high school 2. High school/GED 3. Some college 4. Associate degree 5. Bachelor degree 6. Postgraduate degree	Ordinal	Ordinal Logistic Regression
4a	When I was diagnosed with PE	I didn't believe the doctor/midwife	1. Strongly agree 2. Agree 3. Disagree 4. Strongly disagree 5. Undecided	Ordinal	Ordinal Logistic Regression

Q#	Question	Label (from East et al., 2011)	Response option	Data type	Analysis notes
6d	How my preeclampsia affected my early experience with my baby/babies	It was a shock to know that I might have to give birth early	1. Strongly agree 2. Agree 3. Disagree 4. Strongly disagree 5. Undecided	Ordinal	Ordinal Logistic Regression

Note. PE = preeclampsia

Table 2

Variables and Survey Items From Research Questions

Variable	Dependent/ independent	Level of measurement	Survey items
Research Question 1			
Knowledge of preeclampsia	Dependent	Ordinal/Binary Ratio	3a, 4a, 4c, 4d, 8b,
Demographic characteristics	Independent	Binary Ratio	A, B, C, D, E
Research Question 2			
Attitudes of preeclampsia	Dependent	Ordinal Ratio	5a, 5e, 5f, 9a, 9b
Acculturation	Independent	Ordinal Ratio	8g, 8h, 8i, 8m
Research Question 3			
Perceptions of preeclampsia	Dependent	Binary Ratio	7a, 7b, 8a, 8k
Access to health care	Independent	Ordinal Ratio	4e, 6a, 6c
Research Question 4			
Knowledge of preeclampsia	Dependent	Ordinal/Binary Ratio	3a, 4a, 4c, 4d, 8b
Cultural beliefs	Independent	Binary Ratio	F, H, I, 3a, 3c, 3d, 5b
Research Question 5			
Attitudes ofpreeclampsia	Dependent	Ordinal Ratio	5a, 5e, 5f, 9a, 9b
Socioeconomic status	Independent	Ordinal Ratio	G, 4b, 6b, 7c, 9c, 9e, 9f

Table 3

Experiences

Experience #		Theme	Comment
3		Knowledge	During my pregnancy but before I was diagnosed with preeclampsia.
	3a		I knew about preeclampsia
4		Could not happen	When I was diagnosed with preeclampsia
	4a		I thought it couldn't happen to me
	4c	Not serious	I thought it was not serious or life threatening
	4d	Frightened	I was frightened
	4e	Let self down	I felt a sense of having let myself down by becoming sick with preeclampsia
5		Lost control	As the preeclampsia continued or became more severe.
	5a		I felt that I had lost control of my destiny
	5e	No-one around	I felt that no one around me had been through the same experience as I had
	5f	Realize sick	I did not realize how sick I really was
6		Baby dead	How my preeclampsia affected my early experience with my baby/baby.
	6a		Did your experience of preeclampsia result in the death of your baby?
	6c	Support	Did you feel supported by the hospital staff following your baby's death?
7		Bond Sick	I felt that my ability to initially bond with my baby was limited . . . .
	7a		Because I was too sick
	7b		Because my baby was too sick
8		Counseling	In the weeks, months, or years since my preeclampsia experience . . .
	8a		I have had professional counseling to talk about my experience
	8b	Obtain information	I felt the need to obtain more information about preeclampsia
	8g	Talking helped	I have found that talking about my experience with preeclampsia has helped me

Experience #	Theme	Comment
8h	Confidence	I have had very little confidence in my mothering ability
8i	Self worth	I have had a strong sense of self-worth
8k	Baby care	My baby has needed extra healthcare
8m	Genetic	I have become aware that there may be a genetic link for preeclampsia; for example, my mother had preeclampsia
9	Length pregnancy	We are interested in how your experience of preeclampsia affected later pregnancies
9a		My experience with preeclampsia influenced how long it was between the preeclampsia pregnancy and the next pregnancy
9b	Enjoyment	Enjoyment of the pregnancy

Ethical Considerations

The main concern of this study was the safety and privacy of the participants and the participants' recognition that participation in the study was voluntary. I took the course offered by the National Institutes of Health Office of Extramural Research entitled "Protecting Human Research Participants". All women who accessed the link on the flyer completed the survey that was approved by the Walden University Institutional Review Board (IRB) with the study procedures and instruments prior to beginning recruitment or data collection.

All participants were given equal chance and were aware of the freedom to decline participation at anytime; their decisions were respected. The women did not feel coerced into participating: I used the principle of voluntary participation, which means that women and family members were not coerced into participating in the research. These women accessed the link to imply consent and completed an online survey that they voluntarily agreed to complete after they were made aware of the study design and the involvement needed in the research. Participants were given several opportunities to ask me questions. They were notified that they could withdraw their participation at any point in the study without any penalty or consequence. Participants were not paid for their participation in the study; therefore, remuneration was not a coercing factor influencing study participation (Poly, 2010).

Because the research was conducted online, confidentiality did not pose a problem. For example, information about their gravidity might have revealed something to the participant's husband or another person. The IRB at Walden University protects the researcher from unseen cases that potentially could present an ethical dilemma that could end in legal problems (Trochim, 2006).

This research study was conducted online; therefore, participants did not have any risk of physical harm. Additionally, the risk of mental harm was expected to be low. One potential source of stress for participants was recollecting their experiences with preeclampsia and associated thoughts and beliefs. It is possible that this could be emotionally stressful; however I did not believe there would significant stressors for women and the risks did not warrant the discontinuation of the study or further modifying study procedures. I did not feel the study would significantly impact the risk-benefit ratio of the study. I made every effort to be well informed about cultural, religious, and socioeconomic characteristics of first-generation Nigerian women. The study collaborators were not able to access the completed questionnaires (online data). I made every effort to respect the participants themselves and their privacy, confidentiality, and safety. I adhered to the inclusion and exclusion criteria and did not discriminate against participants in any way.

There may be potential benefits of the research findings to the pregnant first-generation Nigerian women, the Nigerian community, African American women, and Caucasian women in Queens, Brooklyn, the Bronx, and Long Island areas of New York. Also the Preeclampsia Foundation and others with an interest in the issue of preeclampsia, who may make changes to improve the morbidity and mortality rate of preeclampsia as a result of the findings, will be informed of the study findings. There were no external parties' contributions in resources in support of this study. Therefore, no conflicts of interest exist. The findings of the study will be made known to the study participants 4 months after completing the dissertation.

With the approval of Walden University Research Office and Walden University IRB (approval number 09-05-12-0038186, dated September 5, 2012) and the permission of the Nigerian community the next step evolved.

Summary

In chapter 3, the research methodology was discussed as planned. This quantitative study using a cross-sectional survey described the knowledge, attitudes, and perceptions of preeclampsia among 180 participants of first-generation Nigerian women. Detail data of the study to test hypotheses was explained. The survey instrument was a version of East et al questionnaire to be answered by participants online.

Data was collected using BlogSpot Docs online SurveyMonkey and analyzed with SPSS. Logistic regression was used to create odds ratios for each variable and determine the relationship between the independent and dependent variables. Chi-Square test was used to determine statistical significance ($p < 0.05$). Finally this chapter discussed the protection of human subjects and the plan of dissemination of the findings of the research.

CHAPTER 4

Results

Introduction

This study was designed to assess the relationship among the knowledge, attitudes, and perceptions of preeclampsia among first-generation Nigerian women in the United States. Collection of data started on September 8, 2012 and concluded on October 7, 2012.

Following the research methods described in Chapter 3, this chapter describes the data collected from the questionnaire and responds to the research questions. The results of Chapter 4 are divided into (a) demographic description and findings, (b) information of variables used for proportional odds ratios, and (c) summary of the results. Data were collected through SurveyMonkey and analyzed with SPSS 17.0 for descriptive and inferential analysis. The goal of this quantitative, cross-sectional research was to examine and analyze data determining the relationship of knowledge, attitudes, and perceptions among first-generation Nigerian women in the United Statand demographic characteristics, cultural beliefs, technology, acculturation, and access to health care. These were the research questions and hypotheses used:

Research Question 1

Is there a relationship between demographic characteristics, cultural beliefs, socioeconomic status, acculturation, and access to health care and knowledge of preeclampsia among first-generation Nigerian women with a history of preeclampsia living in the United States?

Null hypothesis: There is no relationship between demographic characteristics, cultural beliefs, socioeconomic status, acculturation, and access to health care and knowledge of preeclampsia among first-generation Nigerian women with a history of preeclampsia living in the United States.

Alternative hypothesis: Demographic characteristics, cultural beliefs, socioeconomic status, acculturation, and access to health care will be significantly related to knowledge of preeclampsia among first-generation Nigerian women with a history of preeclampsia living in the United States.

Research Question 2

Is there a relationship between demographic characteristics, cultural beliefs, socioeconomic status, acculturation, and access to health care and attitudes of preeclampsia among first-generation Nigerian women with a history of preeclampsia living in the United States?

Null hypothesis: There is no relationship between demographic characteristics, cultural beliefs, socioeconomic status, acculturation, and access to health care and attitudes of preeclampsia among first-generation Nigerian women with a history of preeclampsia living in the United States.

Alternative hypothesis: Demographic characteristics, cultural beliefs, socioeconomic status, acculturation, and access to health care will be significantly related to attitudes of preeclampsia among first-generation Nigerian women with a history of preeclampsia living in the United States.

Research Question 3

Is there a relationship between demographic characteristics, cultural beliefs, socioeconomic status, acculturation, and access to health care and perceptions of preeclampsia among first-generation

Nigerian women with a history of preeclampsia living in the United States?

Null hypothesis: There is no relationship between demographic characteristics, cultural beliefs, socioeconomic status, acculturation, and access to health care and perceptions of preeclampsia among first-generation Nigerian women with a history of preeclampsia living in the United States.

Alternative hypothesis: Demographic characteristics, cultural beliefs, socioeconomic status, acculturation, and access to health care will be significantly related to perceptions of preeclampsia among first-generation Nigerian women with a history of preeclampsia living in the United States.

Demographic Description of Population and Findings

A purposive sample of first-generation Nigerian women living in the United States was surveyed through the BlogSpot Docs online survey tool. A total of 180 participants were recruited through advertisements that were posted in Nigerian churches, in African markets, and through individual distribution of flyers. Participants were solicted through many sources such as braiding salons, Nigerian churches, grocery stores, physicians' offices, universities, community centers, and word-of-mouth. Demographic data were obtained from a questionnaire from East et al. (2011). Table 4 presents frequency counts and percentages of participants' demographic data.

Table 4

Frequency Counts and Percentages of Participants' Demographic Data

Variables	Frequency	Percentages
Employment status		
Full time	123	68.33
Part time	21	11.67
Unemployed	26	14.44
Other	10	5.56
Total	180	100.00
Maritastatus		
Married	109	60.56
Single	31	17.22
Divorced/separated	31	17.22
Widowed	9	5.00
Total	180	100.00
Educational level		
< High school	10	5.56
High school/GED	26	14.44
College	16	8.89
Associate's degree	100	55.56
Bachelor's degree	28	15.56
Total	180	100.00
WIC		
No	115	63.89
Yes	65	36.11
Total	180	100.00
Health Insurance		
No	31	17.22
Yes	149	82.78
Total	180	100.00

Although the result of the employment of the women was not significant, part-time women were more likely (15%—OR of 1.15) to have the lowest knowledge compare to the full time women. Unemployed women were a little less likely to have lowest response in knowledge versus all other responses (only 4%—unemployed women compared to full time employed women). From full time employment to part- time employment (going from 1 to 2 in employment), the odds of the lowest knowledge (less agreement with knowledge question) versus the combined higher knowledge categories are 1.15. This means, the odds of reporting the lowest knowledge versus the three higher knowledge categories is 1.15 time higher (OR = 1.15, CI = 0.45-2.98) for full time employed women compared to part-time employed women. These results are not statistically significant because the p-value is 0.76. Additionally, because of the proportional odds assumption, one can also say that, for full time employed versus part-time employed women, the odds of reporting the highest knowledge is 1.15 times higher than all lower knowledge categories. For unemployed women versus full time employed women, the odds of reporting the lowest knowledge is 0.96 times greater than the odds for reporting higher knowledge.

For marital status, the odds of reporting the lowest knowledge of preeclampsia was lower than the odds of reporting higher knowledge of preeclampsia, for women who were single (OR = 0.90, 95% CI = 0.40-2.05, p-value 0.40) divorced or separated (OR = 0.71, 95% CI = 0.32- 3.20, p-value is 0.40) or widowed (OR = 0.86, 95% CI = 0.23-3.19, p-value 0.82) compared to being married. For women with health insurance compared to women without health, odds of responding *disagree* are 0.59 times lower (OR = 0.59, CI = 0.28-1.25) than the odds of responding strongly agree or agree. Therefore, the results are not statistically significant.

Employment results were as follows—although no results were significant: part-time employed women were a little more likely (only 15%, because OR is 1.15) to say they had the lowest knowledge (versus all other responses) compared to full-time employed women. Unemployed women were a little less likely (only 4%, because OR is

.96) to say they had the lowest knowledge (versus all other responses) compared to full-time employed women.

For independent variables like WIC and health insurance, *No* is the reference group, so it would be for those with WIC versus those without WIC, or those with insurance versus those without insurance (independent variables always go from lowest category—reference—to highest category). Equally, dependent variables go from lowest category—high agreement—to higher category—lower agreement. The interpretation is in odds ratios from a (binary/dichotomous) logistic regression. The question marital status was recoded as Married 2 for the analyses, which combines divorced and separated into one category for parsimony, and provided married (uncombined) tabulation.

Variables Used in Research Question 1: Analysis and Findings

Ordinal or ordered logistic regression analysis was used. The data were collected on 180 first-generation Nigerian women and organized and analyzed with the results as odds ratio, 95% confidence interval, and $p > |z|$ (*p*-value) columns. In the output, results are displayed as proportional odds ratios. In these results the "reference group" is always the one with stronger agreement: it will either be that of highest agreement or all categories higher than the lowest agreement. Some variables such as *frightened* and *lost contro* were not analyzed because of the small sample size. *Obtain information* and *counseling* also were not used because there were no variations; and *realize sick* and *length of pregnancy* had questionable standard errors; convergence was not achieved. *Enjoyment* was not used because only 1 among 180 participants disagreed.

Knowledge of Preeclampsia

Ordinal logistic regression was conducted to examine the relationship between knowledge of preeclampsia and socioeconomic characteristics, acculturation, and access to health. No statistically significant relationships were found between knowledge of preeclampsia and these characteristics (see Table 5).

Table 5

Knowledge of Preeclampsia: Experiences 3a—I Knew About Preeclampsia

Ordered logistic regression			Number of participants		180	
			LR chi²(3)		0.12	
			Prob > chi²		0.9894	
Log likelihood = -186.02048			Pseudo R^2		0.0003	
					95% Confidence interval	
Knowledge	Odds ratio	Std. error	Z	$P > |z|$	Upper	Lower
_Iemployment-2	1.154	.559	0.30	0.768	.447	2.981
_Iemployment-3	.959	.411	-0.10	0.922	.414	2.219
_Iemployment-4	.947	.597	-0.09	0.931	.276	3.256
/cut1	-1.526	.221			-1.958	-1.094
/cut2	1.464	.218			1.037	1.891
/cut3	2.647	.317			2.027	3.268

Thinking Preeclampsia Could Not Affect Them

No statistically significant relationships were found between thinking that preeclampsia could not affect them and socioeconomic characteristics, acculturation, and access to health. The odds of reporting the lowest versus higher categories of agreement with thinking that preeclampsia could not affect them was 1.26 times higher (OR = 1.26, 95% CI = 0.50-3.12, p-value 0.62) for women who were part-time employed versus full-time employed, 1.27 times higher (OR = 1.27, 95% CI = 0.55-2.97, p-value 0.57) for women who were unemployed versus full-time employed, and 0.94 times lower (OR = 0.94, 95% CI = 0.26-3.43, p-value 0.92) or women who reported other for their employment versus full-time employed women.

I Thought Preeclampsia Was Not Serious or Life Threatening

There was no significance between thinking preeclampsia was not serious or life threatening and the variables. The odds of reporting the lowest versus highest categories of thinking preeclampsia was not serious were 0.8, (OR = 0.8, 95% CI = 0.1-1, p-value 0.81) for women who thought preeclampsia was not serious or life threatening.

Variables Used in Research Question 2: Analysis and Findings

Attitudes of Preeclampsia

Ordinal logistic regression was conducted to examine the relationships between attitudes of preeclampsia and socioeconomic characteristics, acculturation, and access to health.

Felt I Lost Control of My Destiny

No participants reported that they disagreed or strongly disagreed with the item stating that because of preeclampsia they felt they lost control of their destiny. This precluded a proper data analysis on this item.

Felt That No One Around Had the Same Experiences

No participants disagreed or strongly disagreed with the item stating that because of preeclampsia, they felt that no one around had the same experiences. This precluded a proper data analysis on this item. See Table 6 for tabular information from Research Question 1.

Table 6

Tabulation of Themes for Research Question 1

Theme	Frequency	Percent	Cumulative
Knowledge			
a lot |	32	17.78	17.78
a little |	114	63.33	81.11
very little |	22	12.22	93.33
not at all |	12	6.67	100.00
Total	180	100.00	
Could Not Happen			
strongly agree|	104	57.78	57.78
agree|	72	40.00	97.78
disagree|	4	2.22	100.0
Total	180	100.00	
Not Serious			
strongly agree|	142	78.89	78.89
agree|	33	18.33	97.22
disagree|	5	2.78	100.00
Total	180	100.00	
Frightened			
strongly agree|	146	81.11	81.11
agree|	34	18.89	100.00
Total	180	100.00	
Counseling			
Yes|	180	100.00	100.00
Total	180	100.00	

Did Not Realize How Sick I Was

Because of low sample sizes (only one participant responded *strongly disagree* and none responded *disagree*) on the item stating that they did not realize how sick they really were, most regression analyses were not possible. Analyses for reporting getting WIC assistance and having health care are reported in Table 7. The odds of reporting the lowest versus higher categories of agreement about not realizing how sick they were was 0.55 times lower (OR = 0.55, 95% CI = 0.19-1.60, p-value 0.27)for women collecting WIC versus those not on WIC and 1.21 times higher (OR = 1.21, 95% CI = 0.33-4.4, p-value 0.77)for women with health insurance versus those without health insurance. See Table 8 for tabular information from Research Question 2.

Table 7

Realize Sick—Experiences 5f—I Did Not Realize How Sick I Really Was

Ordered logistic regression	Number of participants		180			
	LR chi²(1)		0.09			
	Prob > chi²		0.7689			
Log likelihood = -186.02048	Pseudo R^2		0.0006			
					95% Confidence interval	
Realize sick	Odds ratio	Std. error	Z	$P > |z|$	Upper	Lower
health insurance	1.210	.798	0.29	0.773	0.332	4.407
/cut1	2.239	.607			1.049	3.429
/cut2	5.347	1.149			3.095	7.599

Table 8

Tabulation of Themes for Research Question 2

Theme	Frequency	Percent	Cumulative
Lost Control			
strongly agree|	150	83.33	83.33
agree|	30	16.67	100.00
Total	180	100.00	
No one Around			
strongly agree|	78	43.33	43.33
agree|	99	55.00	98.33
disagree|	3	1.67	100.00
Total	180	100.00	
Realize Sick			
strongly agree|	160	88.89	88.89
agree|	19	10.56	99.44
strongly disagree|	1	0.56	100.00
Total	180	100.00	
Length of pregnancy			
strongly agree|	174	96.67	96.67
agree|	6	3.33	100.00
Total	180	100.00	
Employment			
strongly agree|	144	80.00	80.00
agree|	35	19.44	99.44
strongly disagree|	1	0.56	100.00
Total	180	100.00	

Variables Used in Research Question 3 Analysis and Findings

Ordinal logistic regression was conducted to examine the relationships between perceptions of preeclampsia and socioeconomic characteristics, acculturation, and access to health.

Ability to Bond was Limited Because She was Sick

The odds of reporting the lowest versus higher categories of agreement with feeling that their ability to bond with their baby was limited because the mother was sick was 1.12 times higher (OR = 1.12, 95% CI = 0.46-2.76, p-value 0.80) for women who were part-time employed, 0.96 times lower (OR = 0.96, 95% CI = 0.40-2.32, p-value 0.93) for women who were unemployed, and 1.04 times higher (OR = 1.04, 95% CI = 0.27-3.97, p-value 0.95) for women who reported *other* for their employment, compared to women who were employed full-time (see Table 9).

Table 9

*Bond/Sick: Experiences 7a—Because I Was
Too Sick to Bond With My Baby*

Ordered logistic regression			Number of observations		180		
			LR chi²(3)		0.08		
			Prob > chi²		0.9942		
Log likelihood = -186.02048			Pseudo R^2		0.0002		
						95% Confidence interval	
Bond/sick	Odds ratio	Std. error	Z	$P > \|z\|$	Upper	Lower
_Iemployment-2 |	1.123	.516	0.25	0.800	.456	2.764
_Iemployment-3 |	.964	.433	-0.08	0.935	.400	2.325

_Iemployment~4	1.036	.710	0.05	0.959	.270	3.969
/cut1		.189	.176		-.157	.534
/cut2		2.484	.293		1.909	3.059
/cut3		3.378	.427		2.542	4.215

Ability to Bond Was Limited Because Baby Was Sick

The odds of reporting the lowest versus higher categories of agreement with feeling that their ability to bond with their baby was limited because their baby was sick was 0.43 times lower (OR = 0.43, 95% CI = 0.09-2.11, p-value 0.30)for women who were part-time employed, 0.47 times lower (OR = 0.47, 95% CI = 0.12-1.94, p-value 0.29)or women who were unemployed, and 1.85 times higher (OR = 1.85, 95% CI = 0.28-12.18, p-value 0.5)or women who reported other for their employment, compared to women who were employed full time. See Table 10 for tabular information from Research Question 3.

Table 10

Tabulation of Themes for Research Question 3

Theme	Frequency	Percent	Cumulative
Bond/Sick			
strongly agree|	98	54.44	54.44
agree|	68	37.78	92.22
disagree|	8	4.44	96.67
strongly disagree|	6	3.33	100.00
Total	180	100.00	
Bond Baby Sick			
strongly agree|	3	1.67	1.67
agree|	5	2.78	4.44
disagree|	161	89.44	93.89
strongly disagree|	11	6.11	100.00

Theme	Frequency	Percent	Cumulative
Total	180	100.00	
Obtain Information			
no|	180	100.00	100.00
Total			
Baby Care			
strongly agree|	112	62.22	62.22
agree|	13	7.22	69.44
disagree|	51	28.33	97.78
strongly disagree|	4	2.22	100.00
Total	180	100.00	

Baby Needed Extra Healthcare

The odds of reporting the lowest versus higher categories of agreement with reporting that their baby needed extra healthcare was 1.17 times higher (OR = 1.17, 95% CI = 0.48-2.90, p-value 0.72) for women who were part-time employed, 0.94 times lower (OR = 0.94, 95% CI = 0.39-2.26, p-value 0.88) for women who were unemployed, and 1.04 times higher (OR = 1.04, 95% CI = 0.29-3.71, p-value 0.95) for women who reported other for their employment, compared to women who were employed full ime.

WIC and Health Insurance

The odds of reporting the lowest versus higher categories of agreement with reporting that their baby needed extra healthcare was 0.83 times lower (OR = 0.83, 95% CI = 0.44-1.55) for women collecting WIC versus not on WIC and 0.41 times lower (OR = 0.41, 95% CI = 0.20-0.86) for women with health insurance versus those without health insurance. The association between reporting that their baby needed extra healthcare and reporting that they had health insurance was statistically significant (p = 0.02).

Inferential Analysis

This study used a survey instrument developed by East et al. (2011) and collected demographic data. Responses for the questionnaire addressing knowledge, attitudes, and perceptions of preeclampsia were mixed dichotomous, categorical, continuous, and ordinal, recorded on 5-point Likert-type scale.

Test of Hypothesis

As the dependent variables were ordinal with five levels (or binary), ordinal logistic regressions, based on proportional-odds models, were proposed to investigate the relationships among the dependent variables and the independent variables. Note that if the response variable is binary, then a logistic regression for binary responses was used.

For a binary response variable Y and a vector of independent variables, X, let $\delta(x) = P(\tilde{a} = 1| X = x) = 1 - P(\tilde{a} = 0|X = x)$, where $\delta(x)$ indicates the probability of event $Y = 1$. The logistic regression for $\delta(x) = P(\tilde{a} = 1)$ at values x $= (x_1, \cdots x_p)$ of p predictors could be written as

$$\text{logit } (\pi(x)) = \log \frac{\pi(x)}{1 - \pi(x)} = \alpha + \beta_1 x_1 + \beta_2 x_2 + \cdots + \beta_p x_p. \tag{1}$$

Equation (1) is called the *logit*, the log odds. $\frac{\pi(x)}{1-\pi(x)}$ is called the odds. From Equation (1), the probability of event $Y = 1$, $\delta(x)$, can be derived:

$$\pi(x) = \frac{\exp(\alpha + \beta_1 x_1 + \beta_2 x_2 + \cdots + \beta_p x_p)}{1 + \exp(\alpha + \beta_1 x_1 + \beta_2 x_2 + \cdots + \beta_p x_p)}. \tag{2}$$

The likelihood ratio is used to test the global null hypothesis of all of the $\hat{a}$ being equal to zero. The global null and alternative hypotheses are H0: $\hat{a}_1 = \hat{a}_2 = \cdots = \hat{a}_p = 0$ and Ha: At least one of $\hat{a}_1, \cdots \hat{a}_p$ is not equal to zero.

The Type 3 analysis of effects based on the Wald $\div^2$ test is used to determine if an effect is statistically significant. The null and alternative hypotheses for each effect are

:There is no relationship between the response variable and independent variable X.

Ha: There is a relationship between the response variable and independent variable X.

A *p*-value greater than .05 results in the rejection of the alternate hypothesis; the deviance, Pearson correlation, and Hosmer-Lemeshow goodness-of-fit tests (1, 2, 3) were used to determine the model adequacy (*p*-value > .05 indicates good model fit).

An ordinal logistic regression was proposed to model the relationship between the response variable with five ordered levels (1 = *strongly agree*, 2 = *agree*, 3 = *disagree*, 4 = *strongly disagree*, 5 = *undecided*). The proportional-odds model simultaneously using all cumulative logits is

$$\text{logit}[P(Y \leq j|x)] = \log \frac{P(Y \leq j|x)}{1 - P(Y \leq j|x)} = \alpha_j + \boldsymbol{\beta}^T x. \tag{3}$$

where $j = 1, \ldots, J\text{-}1$. In this case, there are five categories for the response variable (1 = *strongly agree*, 2 = *agree*, 3 = *disagree*, 4 = *strongly disagree*, 5 = *undecided*), so $J = 5, j = 1, \ldots, 4$. $\hat{a}$ is the *p*-dimensional vector of coefficients. Note that what is being modeled is the probability of being in a lower category (1 = strongly agree) in the ordered value list, that is, the probabilities modeled are cumulative over the lower category (1 = strongly agree). Each cumulative logit has its own intercept, a_j, and has the same effects, $\hat{a}$, for each logit. $\mathbf{X}$ is the list of covariates of interest. Hence, the regression coefficients vector, $\hat{a}$, does not depend on j, implying the assumption of the model: The proportional odds model assumes the relationship between $\mathbf{X}$ and Y is independent of j. The validity of the proportional-odds assumption can be checked based on a $\div^2$ score test. An insignificant test result (*p*-value > .05) indicates the proportional-odds assumption is satisfied.

The cumulative-logit model satisfies

$$\text{logit}[P(Y \leq j|x_1)] - \text{logit}[P(Y \leq j|x_2)] = \beta^T(x_1 - x_2). \qquad (4)$$

Similar to the binary logistic regression, the likelihood ratio is used to test the global null hypothesis of all of the $\hat{a}$ being equal to zero. The global null and alternative hypotheses are *H*0: $\hat{a}_1 = \hat{a}_2 = \cdots = \hat{a}_p = 0$ and Ha: At least one of $\hat{a}_1, \cdots \hat{a}_p$ is not equal to zero.

The Type 3 analysis of effects based on the Wald $\div^2$ test is used to determine if an effect is statistically significant. The null and alternative hypotheses for each effect are

*H*0: There is no relationship between the response variable and independent variable *X*.

*H*a: There is a relationship between the response variable and independent variable *X*.

A *p*-value greater than .05 results in the rejection of the alternate hypothesis; the deviance, Pearson correlation, and Hosmer-Lemeshow goodness-of-fit tests (1, 2, 3) were used to determine the model adequacy (*p*-value >.05 indicates good model fit).

Conclusion of Hypothesis

I reject the alternate hypothesis. There is no relationship between demographic characteristics, cultural beliefs, socioeconomic status, acculturation, and access to health careand knowledge, attitudes and perceptions of preeclampsia among first-generation Nigerian women with a history of preeclampsia living in the United States.

Summary of Findings

The results of this study indicate that knowledge, attitudes, and perceptions of preeclampsia are related to socioeconomic status, acculturation, and access to health care. When the response variable (the dependent variable) has more than two categories, ordinal logistic regression (proportional-odds models) was used to investigate the relationship between the dependent variable and independent variables. The results of the present study revealed that the participants were demographically similar. There was some variation in this study, but it was not statistically significant. The interpretation of this last result for health insurance—women who reported lowest agreement (saying their babies did *not* need extra healthcare) were less likely to have healthcare coverage. The opposite direction may be salient for two reasons: (a) women may not feel they need healthcare coverage if they do not have it (perhaps they feel they do not need it), or (b) they did not have coverage, their babies died, so they believed "no, my baby did not need additional coverage, because he/she died."

Chapter 5 includes a summary, interpretation of the findings, social implications of the study, and recommendations for future study and action.

CHAPTER 5

Summary, Conclusion, and Recommendations

Summary

The design of the research study was a cross-sectional survey to assess the relationship among knowledge, attitudes, and perceptions of preeclampsia among 180 first-generation Nigerian living in the United States from the New York area. An online survey was created and participants completed the survey online through a SurveyMonkey questionnaire on a webpage. A quantitative approach and ordinal/binary logistic-regression analysis was used to assess the relationship between independent variables and dependent variables. This particular population was targeted because, although research has provided evidenced of the extent of the disease, a gap existed in understanding the perceptions among first-generation Nigerian women diagnosed with preeclampsia living in the United States. The study population was comprised of 180 first-generation Nigerian women from Queens ($n = 45$), the Bronx ($n = 45$) Brooklyn ($n = 45$), and Long Island ($n = 45$). I administered the online survey to all who accessed the website by implied consent. The data collected enabled a statistical analysis of knowledge, attitudes, and perceptions of preeclampsia based on the questionnaires in the survey. The instrument was developed by East et al. (2011) and I added a demographic questionnaire to attain data structured on a Likert-type scale. The results shown in Chapter 4 were documented as odds ratios, with a 95% confidence interval, and $p > |z|$ (p-value) columns. Prob > ch2 and Pseudo R2, used to determine if the model was good, revealed there was no statistical significance. The Type 3 analysis of effects based on the Wald $\div^2$ test was used to determine if an effect was statistically significant. The null and alternative hypotheses for each effect are H0: There is no relationship between the response variable and independent variable X. Ha: There is a relationship between the response variable and independent variable X. A p-value greater than .05 results in the rejection of the alternate hypothesis. The deviance, Pearson correlation, and Hosmer-Lemeshow goodness-of-fit tests (1, 2, 3) were used to determine the model adequacy (p-value .05 indicates not a good model fit). Chapter 5 will interpret the findings and conclude with a summary, limitations, implications of positive social change, and recommendations.

The Interpretation of Findings

These are the summaries of the research questions and hypotheses:

Research Question 1: Is there a relationship between demographic characteristics, cultural beliefs, socioeconomic status, acculturation, and access to health care and knowledge of preeclampsia among first-generation Nigerian women with a history of preeclampsia living in the United States?

Null hypothesis: There is no relationship between demographic characteristics, cultural beliefs, socioeconomic status, acculturation, and access to health care and knowledge of preeclampsia among first-generation Nigerian women with a history of preeclampsia living in the United States.

Alternative hypothesis: Demographic characteristics, cultural beliefs, socioeconomic status, acculturation, and access to health care will be significantly related to knowledge of preeclampsia among first-generation Nigerian women with a history of preeclampsia living in the United States.

Research Question 2: Is there a relationship between demographic characteristics, cultural beliefs, socioeconomic status, acculturation, and access to health care and attitudes of preeclampsia among first-generation Nigerian women with a history of preeclampsia living in the United States?

Null hypothesis: There is no relationship between demographic characteristics, cultural beliefs, socioeconomic status, acculturation, and access to health care and attitudes of preeclampsia among first-generation Nigerian women with a history of preeclampsia living in the United States.

Alternative hypothesis: Demographic characteristics, cultural beliefs, socioeconomic status, acculturation, and access to health care will be significantly related to attitudes of preeclampsia among first-generation Nigerian women with a history of preeclampsia living in the United States.

Research Question 3: Is there a relationship between demographic characteristics, cultural beliefs, socioeconomic status, acculturation, and access to health care and perceptions of preeclampsia among first-generation Nigerian women with a history of preeclampsia living in the United States?

Null hypothesis: There is no relationship between demographic characteristics, cultural beliefs, socioeconomic status, acculturation, and access to health care and perceptions of preeclampsia among first-generation Nigerian women with a history of preeclampsia living in the United States.

Alternative hypothesis: Demographic characteristics, cultural beliefs, socioeconomic status, acculturation, and access to health care will be significantly related to perceptions of preeclampsia among first-generation Nigerian women with a history of preeclampsia living in the United States.

The results were divided into three separate groups: demographic characteristics, acculturation, and access to health care of first-generation Nigerian women using responses from participants. When the response variable (the dependent variable) had more than two categories, ordinal logistic regression (proportional odds models) was used to investigate the relationship between the dependent variable and independent variables. When the response variable was binary,

binary logistic regression was used. Many respondents did not have prior knowledge of preeclampsia. Those who had prior knowledge indicated their attitude toward preeclampsia was influenced by early detection and follow-up treatment; some indicated that older females in their household downplayed perceptions of preeclampsia.

Analysis Results

Research Question 1: was intended to determine any relationship among demographic characteristics, cultural beliefs, socioeconomic status, acculturation, and access to health care and knowledge of preeclampsia among first-generation Nigerian women with a history of a preeclampsia living in the United States. The results of the regression analysis did not yield a relationship between knowledge of preeclampsia and socioeconomic characteristics, acculturation, access to health, and knowledge of preeclampsia.

Research Question 2: sought to know if there is a relationship among demographic characteristics, cultural beliefs, socioeconomic status, acculturation, and access to health care and attitudes of preeclampsia among first-generation Nigerian women with a history of a preeclampsia living in the United States. The results of the ordinal logistic-regression analysis were not significant and indicated no relationship among the attitudes of preeclampsia and socioeconomic characteristics, acculturation, and access to health care.

Research Question 3: sought to assess whether there is a relationship among demographic characteristics, cultural beliefs, socioeconomic status, acculturation, and access to health care and perceptions of preeclampsia among first-generation Nigerian women with a history of a preeclampsia living in the United States. The result of the ordinal logistic-regression analysis yielded no significance in relationship between the perceptions of preeclampsia and demographic characteristics, acculturation, and access to health care.

Implications for Social Change

This study is important because it identified the gap in knowledge and early detection of preeclampsia to prevent fatality from this disease. Though many pregnant women worldwide suffer from preeclampsia every year, steps to minimize this catastrophe have not yet been effective. A positive social change implication, therefore, created awareness on previously unknown among first-generation Nigerian women with preeclampsia. The new knowledge will achieve by increasingly the broad body of understanding regarding preeclampsia in first-generation Nigerian women living in the United States. There may be an increased understanding of the disease process, bringing awareness of early recognition, and of treatment to decrease disability. This study worked to ensure that women can be healthy in giving birth, free from the complications of preeclampsia. The findings from this study may help move the public health field closer to minimizing complications of preeclampsia among women, thus preventing deaths in pregnancy, labor, and the postpartum period.

The knowledge will be used to educate healthcare providers and the public about the cultural beliefs, attitudes, and perceptions of preeclampsia among first-generation Nigerian women and how these influence healthcare use for early detection and treatment of this disease. The knowledge of the study will help women in the United States better understand how to make positive healthcare decisions, without allowing cultural beliefs, attitudes, and perceptions to influence prospective choices. Knowledge, risk factors, strategies, and educational programs can improve early access to healthcare and follow-up care. The questionnaire responses indicated a need for cultural respect for healthcare-seeking behaviors of first-generation Nigerian women living in the United States to be incorporated into health-assessment programs.

Limitations of the Study

The study focused on a specific target population and in a specific location, potentially influenced by recall bias and inadequate self-reported results. In this study the researcher through exclusive and inclusive criteria addressed the self-reporting bias. The data-collection methods used in this quantitative study determined its structural bias and generalizability. There were many possible variables, but only a subset of them was used to answer the research question. However, these were self-reported cases of preeclampsia with no clinical documentation sought to confirm diagnosis of this illness.

The use of cross-sectional quantitative study did not prove the cause and effect but only demonstrated the relationships of the variables. The quantitative nature of the study, which does not allow for in-depth questioning about pregnancy and personal values, was another limitation. The dependent variable has more than two categories: ordinal logistic regression (proportional odds models) was used to investigate the relationship between the dependent variable and independent variables. When binary logistic regression was used, a problem arose of complete separation or quasicomplete separation; thus, not all the independent variables were included in all models. This research is not statistically significant.

Recommendations for Action

Although the findings are not significant, the findings support the concept that public health departments need to produce a booklet on preeclampsia and distribute it to all healthcare providers regarding the importance of early detection. Additionally, it is necessary to introduce a worldwide educational campaign to educate all women, including grandmothers, mothers, mothers-in-law, and daughters, to bring awareness of preeclampsia. This research study should be disseminated to health department, public healthcare department, healthcare providers, the Nigerian community in New York, and communities in other states. This study can also be disseminated through publication in relevant scientific journals, not for the results but as a new study with social change implications, guidelines for healthcare providers, overview risk factors, complications and positive outcome from early detection of preeclampsia.

Recommendations for Further Studies

There should be additional studies on the education of healthcare providers to seek out women who show early signs of preeclampsia in prenatal clinics, or show early deviation from normal blood pressure and protein in their urine. This study did not compare first-generation Nigerian women living in the United States to Nigerian women living in Nigeria. There should be a study to assess the cultural diet between these two groups and determine any significance. Because cultural attitudes play an important role in the health of many women as to when and how they seek providers when they are pregnant, a study could assess the influence of cultural attitudes. Additional studies should investigate acculturation risk factors among Nigerian women who migrated to the United States. Another recommendation for future studies is to use other methods that will be appropriate to affect the geographical location and recall-bias issues in this purposive study. There should be a study using a qualitative or mixed-methodwith a longitudinal approach and a random selection in a long-term study.

Conclusion

Preeclampsia remains a leading cause of maternal and perinatal mortality and morbidity. Expectant treatment of women with early onset of preeclampsia to improve perinatal outcome should not preclude timely delivery as the key cure (Steegers, von Dadelszen, Duvekot, & Pijnenborg, 2010). Death caused by preeclampsia is avoided with early detection and effective treatment of women with preeclampsia. According to WHO (2011), recommendations maintain a view to promote the best possible clinical practices for the management of preeclampsia.

This study aimed to assess the knowledge, attitudes, and perceptions of first-generation Nigerian women living in the United States. The study indicated evidence that healthcare-seeking behaviors among first-generation Nigerian women are based on knowledge and perceptions of preeclampsia. It is important, therefore, that an awareness of risk factors, clinical manifestation, and treatment modalities be introduced and evaluated periodically on all pregnant women.

References

AbdAlla, S., Lother, H., El Massiery, A., & Quitterer, U. (2001). Increased AT(1) receptor heterodimers in preeclampsia mediate enhanced angiotensin II responsiveness. *Nature Medicine, 9,* 1003-1009. doi:org/10.1038/nm0901-1003

Abubakar, A., Abdullahi, R. A., Jibril, H. Z., Dauda, M. H., & Poopol, M. A. (2009). Maternal ethnicity and severity of pre-eclampsia in northern Nigeria. *Asian Journal of Medical Sciences, 1,* 104-107.

Amburgey, O. A., Chapman, A. C., May, V., Bernstein, I. M., & Cipolla, M. J. (2010). Plasma from preeclamptic women increases blood-brain barrier permeability: Role of vascular endothelial growth factor signaling. *Hypertension, 56,* 1003-1008.

American College of Obstetrics and Gynecology. (2010). New metabolic markers may predict preeclampsia in early pregnancy. *Science Daily.* Retrieved from http://www.sciencedaily.com/releases/2010/09/100913162325.htm

Audibert, F., Boucoiran, I., An, N., Aleksandrov, N., Delvin, E., Bujold, E., & Rey, E. (2010). Screening for preeclampsia using first-trimester serum markers and uterine artery Doppler in nulliparous women. *American Journal of Obstetrics & Gynecology, 203,* 383-388. doi:org/10.1016/j.ajog.2010.06.014

Backes, C. H., Markham, K., Moorehead, P., Cordero, L., Nankervis, C. A., & Giannone, P. J. (2011). Maternal preeclampsia and neonatal outcomes. *Journal of Pregnancy, 2011,* Article ID 214365. doi:10.1155/2011/214365

Bandura, A. (1989). Regulation of cognitive processes through perceived self-efficacy. *Developmental Psychology, 25,* 729-735. do i:org/10.1037/0012-1649.25.5.729

Becker, M. H. (1974). The health belief model and personal health behavior. *Health Education Monographs, 2,* 324-473.

Bellamy, L., Casas, J., Hingorani, A. D., & Williams, D. J. (2007). Pre-eclampsia and risk of cardiovascular disease and cancer in later life: Systematic review and meta-analysis. *British Medical Journal, 335,* 974. doi:org/10.1136/bmj.39335.385301

Bhattacharya, S., & Campbell, D. N. (2005). The incidence of severe complications of pre-eclampsia. *Hypertension in Pregnancy, 24,* 181-190. doi:org/10.1081/PRG-200059873

Biggar, R. J., Poulsen, G., Ng, J., Melbye, M., & Boyd, H. A. (2010). HLA antigen sharing between mother and fetus as a risk factor for eclampsia and preeclampsia. *Human Immunology, 71,* 263-267. doi:org/10.1016/j.humimm.2010.01.006

Bills, V. L., Varet, J., Millar, A., Harper, S. J., Soothill, P. W., & Bates, D. O. (2009). Failure to up-regulate VEGF165b in maternal plasma is a first trimester predictive marker for pre-eclampsia. *Clinical Science, 116,* 265-272. doi:org/10.1042/CS20080270

Blumenstein, M., McMaster, M. T., Black, M. A., Wul, S., Prakash, R., Cooney, J., North, R. A. (2009). A proteomic approach identifies early pregnancy biomarkers for preeclampsia: Novel linkages between a predisposition to preeclampsia and cardiovascular disease. *Proteomics, 9,* 2929-2945. doi:org/10.1002/pmic.200800625

Bonney, E. A. (2007). Preeclampsia: A view through the danger model. *Journal of Reproductive Immunology, 76,* 68-74. doi:org/10.1016/j.jri.2007.03.006

Brichant, G., Dewandre, P. Y., Foidart, J. M., & Brichant, J. F. (2010). Management of severe preeclampsia. *Acta Clinica Belgica, 65*(3), 163-169.

Bridges, E. J., Womble, S., Wallace, M., & McCartney, J. (2003). Hemodynamic monitoring in high-risk obstetrics patients, II: Pregnancy-induced hypertension and preeclampsia. *Critical Care Nurse, 23*(5), 52-57.

Carter, S., & Little, M. (2007). Justifying knowledge, justifying method, taking action: Epistemologies, methodologies, and methods in qualitative research. *Qualitative Health Research, 17,* 1316-1328. doi:org/10.1177/1049732307306927

Centers for Disease Control and Prevention. (2007). Fetal and perinatal mortality, United States, 2004. *National Vital Statistics Reports, 56*(3), 1-19.

Chigbu, C. O., Okezie, O. A., & Odugu, B. U. (2009). Women in southern Nigeria with change in paternity do not have increased incidence of pre-eclampsia. *Journal of Obstetrics and Gynaecology, 29,* 94-97. doi:org/10.1080/01443610802660927

Chikosi, A. B., Moodley, J., Pegoraro, R. J., Lanning, P. A., & Rom, L. (1999). 5, 10 methylenetetrahydrofolate reductase polymorphism in Black South African women with pre-eclampsia. *British Journal of Obstetrics and Gynecology, 106,* 1219-1220.

Cohen, J. (1988). *Statistical power analysis for the behavioral sciences* (2nd ed.). Hillsdale, NJ: Lawrence Erlbaum.

Cooper, C. F., & Lawler, F. H. (2001). Physician perceptions regarding competence of obstetrical providers and attitudes about other issues in obstetrical care. *Journal of the Oklahoma State Medical Association, 94,* 554-560.

Craici, L., Wagner, S., & Garovic, V. D. (2008). Review: Preeclampsia and future cardiovascular risk: Formal risk factor or failed stress test? *Therapeutic Advances in Cardiovascular Disease, 2*(4), 249-259. doi:org/10.1177/1753944708094227

Creinin, M. D., & Simhan, H. N. (2009). Can we communicate gravidity and parity better? *Obstetrics & Gynecology, 113,* 709-711.

Creswell, J. W. (2002). *Educational research: Planning, conducting and evaluating quantitative and qualitative research.* Upper Saddle River, NJ: Merrill/Pearson.

Creswell, J. W. (2003). *Research design qualitative, quantitative, and mixed methods approaches* (2nd ed.). Thousand Oaks, CA: Sage.

Creswell, J. W. (2007). *Qualitative inquiry and research design. Choosing among five approaches* (2nd ed.). Thousand Oaks, CA: Sage.

Dallas Researchers. (2004, April 20). *Understanding preeclampsia in Black women: More folic acid may be needed, study finds.* Retrieved from http://www.msnbc.msn.com

De Ferranti, S. D., Gauvreau, K., Ludwig, D. S., Neufeld, E. J., Newburger, J. W., & Rifai, N. (2004). Prevalence of the metabolic syndrome in American adolescents: Findings from the third national health and nutrition examination survey. *Circulation, 110,* 2494-2497. doi:org/10.1161/01.CIR.0000145117.40114.C7

Denison, J. (1996). *Behavior change—A summary of four major theories.* Retrieved from http://pdf.usaid.gov/pdf_docs/PNABZ712.pdf

Devarajan, P. (2008). *Oliguria.* Retrieved from http://emedicine. medscape.com/article/983156-overview

Dissanayake, V. H. W. (2004). *Inherited factors in pre-eclampsia: Molecular genetics and epidemiological studies in a Sri Lankan population* (Doctoral dissertation). University of Nottingham, Nottingham, UK. Retrieved from http://etheses.nottingham. ac.uk/66/1/vhwdthesis.pdf

Dorland, J. (2010). *Fetal behaviour in preeclamptic compared to low-risk, normotensive pregnancies* (Master's thesis). Available from ProQuest Dissertations & Theses database. (AAT MR44436)

Dragun, D., & Haase-Fielitz, A. (2009). Low catechol-*O*-methyltransferase and 2-methoxyestradiol in preeclampsia: More than a unifying hypothesis. *Nephrology Dialysis Transplantation, 24,* 31-33. doi:org/10.1093/ndt/gfn534

East, C., Conway, K., Pollock, W., Frawley, N., & Brennecke, S. (2011). Women's experiences of preeclampsia: Australian action on preeclampsia survey of women and their confidants. *Journal of Pregnancy,* Article 375653. doi:10.1155/2011/375653

Finn, R. (2005). Preeclampsia presentation varies depending on race and ethnicity. *Obstetrics & Gynecology News.* Retrieved from http://www.encyclopdia.com/OB+GYN+NEWS/publications. aspx?date=200503&pageNumber=1

Fisk, N., & Atun, R. (2009). Systematic analysis of research underfunding in maternal and perinatal health. *BJOG, 116,* 347-356. doi:10.1111/j.1471-0528.2008.02027.x

Gangaram, R., Ojwang, P. J., Moodley, J., & Maharaj, D. (2005). The accuracy of urine dipsticks as a screening test for proteinuria in hypertensive disorders of pregnancy. *Hypertension in Pregnancy, 24*(2), 117-123. doi:org/10.1081/PRG-200059849

Gaufberg, S. V. (2011). *Emergent management of abruptio placentae.* Retrieved from http://emedicine.medscape.com/article/795514-overview

Glanz, K., Rimer, B. K., & Lewis, F. M. (1997). *Health behavior and health education: Theory, Research and Practice.* San Francisco, CA: Wiley & Sons.

Grol, R. (2001). Improving the quality of medical care: Building bridges among professional pride, payer profit, and patient satisfaction. *Journal of the American Medical Association, 286,* 2578-2585. doi:org/10.1001/jama.286.20.2578

Hall, D. R. (2007). Is preeclampsia less common in patients with HIV/AIDS? *Journal of Reproductive Immunology, 76,* 75-77. doi:org/10.1016/j.jri.2007.04.005

Hira, B., Pegoraro, R., Rom, L., & Moodley, J. (2003). Absence of factor V Leiden, thrombomodulin and prothrombin gene variants in Black South African women with pre-eclampsia and eclampsia. *BJOG, 110,* 327-328. doi:org/10.1046/j.1471-0528.2003.01090.x

Hladunewich, M., Karumanchi, S. A., & Lafayette, R. (2007). Pathophysiology of the clinical manifestations of preeclampsia. *Clinical Journal of American Society of Nephrology, 2,* 543-549. doi:10.2215/CJN.03761106

Hofmeyr, G. J., Lawrie, T. A., Atallah, A. N., & Duley, L. (2010). *Calcium supplementation during pregnancy for preventing hypertensive disorders and related problems.* Oxfordshire, UK: The Cochrane Library. doi:10.1002/14651858.CD001059.pub3

Huria, A., Gupta, P., Kumar, D., & Sharma, M. (2010). Vitamin C and vitamin E supplementation in pregnant women at risk for pre eclampsia: A randomized controlled trial. *The Internet Journal of Health, 10*(2). Retrieved from http://www.ispub.com

Idogun, E., Imarengiaye, C., & Momoh, S. (2007). Extracellular calcium and magnesium in preeclampsia and eclampsia. *African Journal of Reproductive Health, 11*(2), 80-85. doi:org/10.2307/25549719

Igberase, G. O., & Ebeigbe, P. N. (2006). Eclampsia: Ten years of experience in a rural tertiary hospital in the Niger Delta, Nigeria. *Journal of Obstetrics & Gynecology, 26*, 414-417. doi: org/10.1080/01443610600720113

Ingec, M., Borekci, B., & Kadanali, S. (2005). Elevated plasma homocysteine concentrations in severe preeclampsia and eclampsia. *The Journal of Clinical Nutrition, 81*, 1390-1396.

Institute of Medicine, Committee for the Study of the Future of Public Health. (1988). *The future of public health.* Washington, DC: National Academy Press.

Janakiraman, V., Gantz, M., Maynard, S., & El-Mohandes, A. (2009). Association of cotinine levels and preeclampsia among African-American women. *Nicotine Tobacco Research, 11*, 679-684. doi:org/10.1093/ntr/ntp049

Jim, B., Sharma, S., Kebede, T., & Acharya, A. (2010). Hypertension in pregnancy. *Cardiology in Review, 18*, 178-189. doi:org/10.1097/CRD.0b013e3181c60ca6

Johnson, S. S., Driskell, M. M., Johnson, J. L., Prochaska, J. M., Zwick, W., & Prochaska, J. O. (2006). Efficacy of a transtheoretical model-based expert system for antihypertensive adherence. *Disease Management, 9*(5), 291-301. doi:org/10.1089/dis.2006.9.291

Kaaja, R. J., Moore, M. P., Yandle, T. G., Ylikorkala, O., Frampton, C. M., & Nicholls, M. G. (2004). Effect of changes in body posture on vasoactive hormones in pre-eclamptic women. *Journal of Human Hypertension, 18*, 789-794._doi:org/10.1038/sj.jhh.1001743

Kanagasabai, S. (2010). Biochemical markers in the prediction of pre-eclampsia: Are we there yet? *The Internet Journal of Gynecology and Obstetrics, 14*(1). Retrieved from http://www.ispub.com

Kanayama, N. (2003). Trophoblastic injury: New etiological and pathological concept of preeclampsia. *Croatian Medical Journal, 44,* 148-156.

Karanam, V. L., Page, M. N., & Anim-Nyame, N. (2010). Hypoxia in pre-eclampsia: Cause or effect? *Current Women's Health Reviews, 6,* 303-308. doi:10.2174/157340410793362131

Karumanchi, S. A., Maynard, S., Sukhatme, V. P., Stillman, I. E., & Epstein, F. H. (2005). Preeclampsia: A renal perspective. *Kidney International, 67,* 2101-2113. doi:10.1111/j.1523-1755.2005.00316.x

Khan, F. (2010). *An evaluation of magnesium status and inflammatory response during the third trimester of normal pregnancy and preeclampsia* (Doctoral dissertation). Available from ProQuest Dissertations & Theses database. (AAT 3322540)

Khan, K., Wojdyla, D., Say, L., Gülmezoglu, A., & Van Look, P. (2006). WHO analysis of causes of maternal death: A systematic review. *The Lancet, 367,* 1066-1074. doi:org/10.1016/S0140-6736(06)68397-9

Kim, Y. J., Park, H., Lee, H. Y., Ahn, Y. M., Ha, E. H., Suh, S. H., & Pang, M. G. (2007). Paraoxonase gene polymorphism, serum lipid, and oxidized low-density lipoprotein in preeclampsia. *European Journal of Obstetrics & Gynecology and Reproductive Biology, 133,* 47-52. doi:org/10.1016/j.ejogrb.2006.07.046

Koopmans, C., Bijlenga, D., Groen, H., Vijgen, S., Aarnoudse, J., Bekedam, D., van Pampus, M. G. (2009). Induction of labour versus expectant monitoring for gestational hypertension or mild pre-eclampsia after 36 weeks gestation (HYPITAT): A multicentre, open-label randomized controlled trial. *The Lancet, 374,* 979-988. doi:org/10.1016/S0140-6736(09)60736-4

Kulkarni, A., Mehendale, S., Pisal, h., Kilari, A., Dangat, K., Salunkhe, S., Joshi, S. (2010). Association of omega-3 fatty acids and homocysteine concentrations in pre-eclampsia. *Clinical Nutrition, 30,* 60-64. doi:org/10.1016/j.clnu.2010.07.007

Lain, K. Y., & Roberts, J. M. (2002). Contemporary concepts of the pathogenesis and management of preeclampsia. *Journal of American Medical Association, 287,* 3183-3186. doi:org/10.1001/jama.287.24.3183

LaMarca, B. D., Gilbert, J., & Granger, J. P. (2008). Recent progress toward the understanding of the pathophysiology of hypertension during preeclampsia. *Hypertension, 51,* 982-988. doi:10.1161/HYPERTENSIONAHA.107.108837

Lennon, J. L. (2005). The use of the health belief model in Dengue health education. *Dengue Bulletin, 29,* 217-219.

Leshem, S., & Trafford, V. (2007). Overlooking the conceptual framework. *Innovations in Education & Teaching International, 44,* 93-105. doi:org/10.1080/14703290601081407

Levine, R. J., & Lindheimer, M. D. (2009). First-trimester prediction of hypertensive disorders in pregnancy. *Hypertension,* 53(5), 747-748. doi:org/ 10.1161/HYPERTENSIONAHA.109.129379

Levine, R. J., Maynard, S. E., Qian, C., Lim, K. H., England, L. J., Yu, K. F., Karumanchi, S. A. (2004). Circulating angiogenic factors and the risk of preeclampsia. *The New England Journal of Medicine, 350,* 672-683. doi:org/10.1056/NEJMoa031884

Levine, R. J., Vatten, L. J., Horowitz, G. L., Qian, C., Romundstad, P. R., Yu, K. F., Karumanchi, S. A. (2009). Preeclampsia, soluble fms-like tyrosine kinase 1, and the risk of reduced thyroid function: Nested case-control and population based study. *British Medical Journal, 339,* b4336. doi:10.1136/bmj.b4336

Li, W., Tang, L., Wu, T., Zhang, J., Liu, G. J., & Zhou, L. (2009). *Chinese herbal medicines for treating pre-eclampsia.* Oxfordshire, UK: The Cochrane Library. doi:10.1002/14651858.CD005126.pub2

Lim, K., & Steinberg, G. (2010, August). *Preeclampsia.* Retrieved from http://emedicine.medscape.com/article/1476919-overview

Lindgren, P., Cederholm, M., Haglund, B., & Axelsson, O. (2010). Invasive procedures for fetal karyotyping: No cause of subsequent gestational hypertension or pre-eclampsia. *BJOG, 117,* 1422-1425. doi:org/10.1111/j.1471-0528.2010.02665.x

López-Pulles, R., González-Andrade, F., Durán-Rodas, M., Ayala, J., Carrillo, R., Buitrón, L. R., . . . Moya, W. (2010). Assessment of genetic contributions to risk of preeclampsia in Ecuadorian women. *Hypertension in Pregnancy, 29,* 410-418. doi :org/10.3109/10641950903572258

Luppi, P., & DeLoia, J. A. (2006). Monocytes of preeclamptic women spontaneously synthesize pro-inflammatory cytokines. *Clinical Immunology, 118,* 268-275. doi:org/10.1016/j.clim.2005.11.001

Makrides, M., Duley, L., & Olsen, S. F. (2007). *Marine oil, and other prostaglandin precursor, supplementation for pregnancy uncomplicated by pre-eclampsia or intrauterine growth restriction.* Oxfordshire, UK: The Cochrane Library. doi:10.1002/14651858.CD003402. pub2

Manongi, R. N., Marchant, T. C., & Bygbjerg, I. C. (2006). Improving motivation among primary healthcare workers in Tanzania: A health worker perspective. *Human Resources for Health, 4*(6), 1-7. doi:org/10.1186/1478-4491-4-6

Maynard, S. E., Moore S., Bur, L., Crawford, S. L., Solitro, M. J., & Meyer, B. A. (2010). Soluble endoglin for the prediction of preeclampsia in a high risk cohort. *Hypertension in Pregnancy, 29,* 330-341. doi:org/10.3109/10641950902968684

Meher, S., & Duley, L. (2009). *Rest during pregnancy for preventing pre-eclampsia and its complications in women with normal blood pressure.* Oxfordshire, UK: The Cochrane Library. doi:10.1002/14651858. CD005939

Mignini, L. E., Latthe, P. M., Villar, J., Kilby, M. D., Carroli, G., & Khan, K. S. (2005). Mapping the theories of preeclampsia: The role of homocysteine. *American College of Obstetricians and Gynecologists, 105,* 411-425.

Milne, F., Redman, C., Walker, J., Baker, P., Bradley, J., Cooper, C., Waugh, J. (2005). The preeclampsia community guideline (PRECOG): How to screen for and detect onset of preeclampsia in the community. *British Medical Journal, 330,* 576-580. doi:org/10.1136/bmj.330.7491.576

Mulla, Z. D., Gonzalez-Sanchez, J. L., & Nuwayhid, B. (2007). Descriptive and clinical epidemiology of preeclampsia and eclampsia in Florida. *Ethnicity and Disease, 17,* 736-741.

Munger, M. A., Van Tassell., B. W., & LaFleur, L. (2007). Medication nonadherence: An unrecognized cardiovascular risk factor. *Medscape General Medicine, 9*(3), 58.

Nabili, S. (2009). What is thrombocytopenia? *MedicineNet.* Retrieved from http://www.medicinenet.com/thrombocytopenia_low_platelet_count/article.htm

National Center for Biotechnology Information. (2010). Hydatidiform mole; Molar pregnancy. *PubMed Health.* Retrieved from http://www.ncbi.nlm.nih.gov/pubmedhealth/PMH0001907/

National Institute of Child Health. (2005). *Substances found in blood may predict development of preeclampsia.* Retrieved from http://www.nichd.nih.gov/news/releases/preeclampsia.cfm

Nicolaides, K. H., Bindra, R O., Turan, M., Chefetz, I., Sammar, M., Meiri, H., Cuckle, H. S. (2006). A novel approach to first-trimester screening for early pre-eclampsia combining serum PP-13 and Doppler ultrasound. *Ultrasound in Obstetrics & Gynecology, 27*(1), 13-17. doi:org/10.1002/uog.2686

Nwosu, Z., & Omabe, M. (2010). Maternal and fetal consequences of preeclampsia. The *Internet Journal of Gynecology and Obstetrics, 13*(1). Retrieved from http://www.ispub.com

Okafor, U. V., Efetie, E. R., Igwe, W., & Okezie, O. (2009). Anaesthetic management of patients with pre-eclampsia/eclampsia and perinatal outcome. *Journal of Maternal Fetal Neonatal Medicine, 22,* 688-692. doi:org/10.1080/14767050902994473

Okafor, U. V., & Ezegwui, H. (2010). Cesarean delivery in preeclampsia and seasonal variation in a tropical rainforest belt. *Journal of Postgraduate Medicine, 56,* 21-23. doi:org/10.4103/0022-3859.62431

Olopade, F. E., & Lawoyin, T. O. (2008). Maternal mortality in a Nigerian maternity hospital. *African Journal of Biomedical Research, 11,* 267-273.

Osungbade, K. O., & Ige, O. K. (2011). Public health perspectives of preeclampsia in developing countries: Implication for health system strengthening. *Journal of Pregnancy,* Article ID 481095. doi:10.1155/2011/481095

Patrick T. E., Powers, R. W., Daftary, A. R., Ness, R. B., & Roberts, J. M. (2004). Homocysteine and folic acid are inversely related in Black women with preclampsia. *Hypertension, 43,* 1279-1282. doi:org/10.1161/01.HYP.0000126580.81230.da

Pérez-Mutul, J., González-Herrera, L., Sosa-Cabrera, T., & Martínez-Olivares, R. (2004). A mutation in the 5, 10-methylenetetrahydrofolate reductase gene is not associated with preeclampsia in women of southeast Mexico. *Archives of Medical Research, 35,* 231-234.

Poly, C. (2010). *Guidelines for human subjects research protocol.* Retrieved from http://www.calpoly.edu/~RGP/policyHS.html

Powers, R. W., Catov, J. M., Bodnar, L. M., Gallaher, M. J., Lain, K. Y., & Roberts, J. M. (2008). Evidence of endothelial dysfunction in preeclampsia and risk of adverse pregnancy outcome. *Reproductive Sciences, 15,* 374-381. doi:10.1177/1933719107311780

Prahlow, J. A., & Barnard, J. J. (2004). Pregnancy-related maternal deaths. *American Journal of Forensic Medicine and Pathology, 25,* 220-236. doi:org/10.1097/01.paf.0000136445.54246.10

Rani, N., Dhingra, R., Arya, D. S., Kalaivani, M., Bhatla, N., & Kumar, R. (2010). Role of oxidative stress markers and antioxidants in the placenta of preeclamptic patients. *Journal of Obstetrics and Gynecology Research, 36,* 1189-1194. doi:org/10.1111/j.1447-0756.2010.01303.x

Rawashdeh, R. (2010). *A systematic review and meta-analysis of genetic associations with preeclampsia* (Unpublished master's thesis). Sarah Lawrence College, Bronxville, NY.

Redman, C. W., & Sargent, I. L. (2005). Latest advances in understanding preeclampsia. *Science, 308,* 1592-1594. doi:org/10.1126/science.1111726

Roberts, J. M., & Gammill, H. S. (2005). Preeclampsia: Recent insights. *Hypertension, 46,* 1243-1249. doi:org/10.1161/01.HYP.0000188408.49896.c5

Rosenstock, I. M. (2005). Why people use health services. *The Milbank Quarterly, 83*(4), 1-32. doi:org/10.1111/j.1468-0009.2005.00425.x

Rosenstock, I. M., Strecher, V. J., & Becker, M. H. (1988). Social learning theory and health belief model. *Health Education Quarterly, 15,* 175-183. doi:org/10.1177/109019818801500203

Ruano, R., Fontes, R. S., & Zugaib, M. (2005). Prevention of preeclampsia with low-dose aspirin—A systematic review and meta-analysis of the main randomized controlled trials. *Clinics (Sao Paulo), 60,* 407-414. doi:org/10.1590/S1807-59322005000500010

Sanchez, S. E., Zhang, C., Malinow, M. R., Ware-Jauregui, S., Larrabure, G., & Williams, M. A. (2001). Plasma folate, vitamin B12, and homocyst(e)ine concentrations in preeclamptic and normotensive Peruvian women. *American Journal of Epidemiology, 153,* 474-480. doi:org/10.1093/aje/153.5.474

SAS Institute Inc. (2012). *SAS/STAT 9.3 user's guide* (2nd ed.). Cary, NC: SAS Institute.

Savvidou, M., Akolekar, R., Zaragoza, E., Poon, L., & Nicolaides, K. (2009). First trimester urinary placental growth factor and development of pre-eclampsia. *International Journal of Obstetrics and Gynecology, 116,* 643-647.

Sebire, N. J., Fox, H., Backos, M., Rai, R., Paterson, C., & Regan, L. (2002). Defective endovascular trophoblast invasion in primary antiphospholipid antibody syndrome-associated early pregnancy failure. *Human Reproduction, 17,* 1067-1071. doi:org/10.1093/humrep/17.4.1067

Semenovskaya, Z., & Erogul, M. (2010). *Pregnancy, preeclampsia.* Retrieved from http://danilatos.wordpress.com/2010/07/17/preeclampsia/

Shaarawy, M., Zaki, S., Ramzi, A., Salem, M. E., & El-Minawi, A. M. (2005). Feto-maternal bone remodeling in normal pregnancy and preeclampsia. *Journal of the Society for Gynecologic Investigation, 12,* 343-348. doi:org/10.1016/j.jsgi.2005.02.014

Shenoy, V., Kanasaki, K., & Kalluri, R. (2010). Pre-eclampsia: Connecting angiogenic and metabolic pathways. *Trends in Endocrinology and Metabolism, 21,* 529-536._doi:org/10.1016/j.tem.2010.05.002

Sibai, B. M. (2004). Diagnosis, controversies, and management of the syndrome of hemolysis, elevated liver enzymes, and low platelet count. *Obstetrics & Gynecology, 103,* 981-991. doi:org/10.1097/01.AOG.0000126245.35811.2a

Sibai, B. M., & Stella, C. L. (2010). Diagnosis and management of atypical preeclampsia-eclampsia. *Obstetric Anesthesia Digest, 30,* 12-13. doi:org/10.1097/01.aoa.0000366992.20321.da

Siddiqui, S., Goodman, N., McKenna, S., Goldie, M., Waugh, J., & Brightling, C. (2008). Pre-eclampsia is associated with airway hyperresponsiveness. *International Journal of Obstetrics and Gynecology, 115,* 520-522.

Skjaerven R., Vatten L. J., Wilcox A. J., Ronning, T., Irgens L. M., & Lie R. T. (2005) Recurrence of preeclampsia across generations: Exploring fetal and maternal genetic components in a population based cohort. *British Medical Journal, 331,* 877. doi:10.1136/bmj.38555.462685.8F

Smith, G. C., Stenhouse, E. J., Crossley, J. A., Aitken, D. A., Cameron, A. D., & Connor, M. J. (2002). Early pregnancy levels of pregnancy-associated plasma protein A and the risk of intrauterine growth restriction, premature birth, preeclampsia, and stillbirth. *Journal of Clinical Endocrinology & Metabolism, 87,* 1762-1767. doi:org/10.1210/jc.87.4.1762

Soemarno, (2007). *Quantitative and quantitative research.* Retrieved from http://www.slideshare.net/guest3bd2a12/quantitative-research-presentation

Spaanderman, M. E., Ekhart, T. H., de Leeuw, P. W., & Peeters, L. L. (2004). Angiotensin II sensitivity in nonpregnant formerly preeclamptic women and healthy parous controls. *Journal of the Society for Gynecologic Investigation, 11,* 416-422. doi:org/10.1016/j.jsgi.2004.06.003

Srinivas, S. K., Edlow, A. G., Neff, M. P., Sammel, M. D., Andrela, C. M., & Elovitz, M. A. (2009). Rethinking IUGR in preeclampsia: Dependent or independent of maternal hypertension? *Journal of Perinatology, 29,* 680-684. doi:org/10.1038/jp.2009.83

Steegers, E. A., von Dadelszen, P., Duvekot, J. J., & Pijnenborg, R. (2010). Pre-eclampsia. *The Lancet, 376,* 631-644. doi:10.1016/SO140-6736(10)60279-6

Swende, T., & Abwa, T. (2009). Reversible blindness in fulminating preeclampsia. *Annals of African Medicine, 8,* 189-191.

Thadhani, R., & Solomon, C. (2008). Preeclampsia—A glimpse into the future? *The New England Journal of Medicine, 359,* 858-860. doi:org/10.1056/NEJMe0804637

Topal, G., Foudi, N., Uydes-Dogan, B. S., Cachina, T., Kucor, M., Gezer, A.Norel, X. (2010). Involvement in prostaglandin F2a in preeclamptic human umbilical vein vasospasm: A role of prostaglandin F and thromboxane A2 receptors. *Journal of Hypertension, 28,* 2438-2445.

Trochim, W. M. K. (2006). Ethics in research. *Research Methods Knowledge Base.* Retrieved from http://www.socialresearchmethods.net/kb/ethics.php

Tucker, M. J., Berg, C. J., Callaghan, W. M., & Hsia, J. (2007). The Black-White disparity in pregnancy-related mortality from 5 conditions: Differences in prevalence and case-fatality rates. *American Journal of Public Health, 97,* 247-251. doi:org/10.2105/AJPH.2005.072975

Uboh, F. E., Ebong, P. E., Oton, E., Itam I. H., &. Barnaby, N. (2008). Antioxidant vitamins and free radical status in Nigerian pre-eclamptic women. *Research Journal of Obstetrics & Gynecology, 1,* 30-33. doi:org/10.3923/rjog.2008.30.33

Ulin, P. R., Robinson, E. T., & Tolley, E. E. (2005). *Qualitative methods in public health: A field guide for applied research.* San Francisco, CA: Jossey-Bass.

Vallotton, C. D. (2008). Signs of emotion: What can preverbal children "say" about internal states? *Infant Mental Health Journal, 29,* 234-258. doi:org/10.1002/imhj.20175

Van der Merwe, J. L., Hall, D. R., Wright, C., Schubert, P., & Grove, D. (2010). Are early and late preeclampsia distinct subclasses of the disease—What does the placenta reveal? *Hypertension Pregnancy, 29,* 457-467. doi:org/10.3109/10641950903572282

Vigeh, M., Yokoyama, K., Ramezanzadeh, F., Dahaghin, M., Sakai, T., Morita, Y., Kobayashi, Y. (2006). Lead and other trace metals in preeclampsia: A case-control study in Tehran, Iran. *Environmental Research, 100,* 268-275. doi:org/10.1016/j.envres.2005.05.005

Vigil-De Gracia, P., Montufar-Rueda, C., & Ruiz, J. (2003). Expectant management of severe preeclampsia and preeclampsia superimposed on chronic hypertension between 24 and 34 weeks' gestation. *European Journal of Obstetrics & Gynecology and Reproductive Biology, 107,* 24-27. doi:org/10.1016/S0301-2115(02)00269-5

Vitoratos, N., Economou, E., Iavazzo, C., Panoulis, K., & Creatsas, G. (2010). Maternal serum levels of TNF-Alpha and IL-6 long after delivery in preeclamptic and normotensive pregnant women. *Mediators of Inflammation,* Article ID 908649. doi:10.1155/2010/908649

Wagner, L. K. (2004). Diagnosis and management of preeclampsia. *American Family Physician, 70,* 2317-2324.

Wallenburg, H. C., Dekker, G. A., Makovitz, J. W., & Rotmans, N. (1991). Effect of low-dose aspirin on vascular refractoriness in angiotensin-sensitive primigravid women. *American Journal of Obstetrics & Gynecology, 164,* 1169-1173.

Wilson, J. G. (2009). *Factors affecting heart attack treatment-seeking delay among African American women* (Doctoral dissertation) Walden University. Available from ProQuest Dissertations and Theses database. UMI: 3380357

Woisetschläger, C., Waldenhofer, U., Bur, A., Herkner, H., Kiss, H., Binder, M., Hirschi, M. M. (2000). Increased blood pressure response to the cold pressor test in pregnant women developing pre-eclampsia. *Journal of Hypertension, 18,* 399-403. doi: org/10.1097/00004872-200018040-00007

World Health Organization. (2011). *Recommendations for prevention and treatment of preeclampsia and eclampsia.* Retrieved from www. who.int/reproductivehealth/publications/maternal_perinatal_health/9789241548335/en/index.html

Xiong, X., Demianczuk, N. N., Saunders, L. D., Wang, F., & Fraser, W. D. (2002). Impact of preeclampsia and gestational hypertension on birth weight by gestational age. *American Journal of Epidemiology, 15,* 203-209. doi:org/10.1093/aje/155.3.203

Yeo, S., Wells, P. J., Kieffer, E. C., & Nolan, G. H. (2007). Preeclampsia among Hispanic women in a Detroit health system. *Ethnicity and Disease, 17,* 118-121. doi:org/10.1093/aje/155.3.203

Zeeman, G. G., Fleckenstein, J. L., Twickler, D. M., & Cunningham, F. G. (2004). Cerebral infarction in eclampsia. *American Journal of Obstetrics & Gynecology, 190,* 714-720. doi:org/10.1016/j.ajog.2003.09.015

www.ingramcontent.com/pod-product-compliance
Lightning Source LLC
Chambersburg PA
CBHW050400290526
45786CB00003B/1065